Dear Reader,

Most people take bladder and bowel control for granted—until something goes wrong. Then, unexpectedly, they find themselves hurrying to get to a bathroom on time, avoiding certain situations for fear of leakage, or relying on absorbent pads for protection. If you have had any of these experiences, you are not alone.

An estimated 32 million adults have incontinence, the unintended loss of urine or feces that is significant enough to make it difficult for them to maintain good hygiene and carry on ordinary social and work lives. What's the cause? For women, it's typically a rarely discussed but common result of childbirth and aging. For men, it's most often a side effect of treatment for prostate problems.

Besides disrupting daily activities and nighttime sleep, incontinence can also chip away at your health. If you have stopped exercising for fear of leakage, for example, you are giving up one of the most effective strategies for maintaining health. In addition, getting up several times a night can lead to sleep deprivation and raises the risk of injury from falls. And incontinence that causes withdrawal from social interactions can contribute to depression.

Even more alarming, older women who frequently must rush to the bathroom are 26% more likely to fall and 34% more likely to break a bone. Incontinence is also a leading cause of nursing home placement, and that prospect drives some people to try to hide their condition rather than seek help.

The good news is that treatments are becoming more effective and less invasive. For example, today's medications for urinary incontinence are easier to use than earlier ones. Exercises can help strengthen the muscles of the pelvic floor, shoring up those that control both bladder and bowel. Surgical options include less invasive outpatient procedures that can work as well as older, open surgical procedures.

Although incontinence can engender fear and embarrassment, rest assured that it is not a psychological problem or a personal failure. Incontinence is a medical symptom, and it deserves the same attention you would give to any other medical problem. This report describes the common causes of urinary and fecal incontinence for men and women and the treatments for these conditions.

Sincerely,

May M. Wakamatsu, M.D.
Medical Editor

Joseph A. Grocela, M.D.
Medical Editor

Liliana Bordeianou, M.D.
Medical Editor

Harvard Health Publications | Harvard Medical School | 10 Shattuck Street, Second Floor | Boston, MA 02115

Urinary incontinence

In the United States, an estimated 18 million people have daily urinary incontinence, and another 34 million feel the need to urinate with increasing urgency and frequency but manage to avoid accidents. Because damage sustained during vaginal childbirth is a major cause of incontinence, the problem is much more common in women—estimates go as high as 32% in older women. Men are less commonly affected—5% to 15%, according to government estimates—but the rates are increasing as more men undergo surgery or other treatments of the prostate gland (see Figure 1). More than half of nursing home residents have urinary incontinence. Incontinence may also be related to an underlying medical condition, treatment, or injury.

Incontinence is costly. Every year, Americans spend about $19.5 billion coping with urinary incontinence, and an additional $12.6 billion on urinary urgency and frequency. Of that total, most goes toward managing the condition or its complications rather than toward diagnosis and treatment. If you are coping with incontinence, you understand all too well the high cost of pads and special absorbent clothing. Add to this the cost of treatment, lost work time, and the emotional toll this condition extracts, and the price is high indeed.

Anatomy of urinary continence

The job of your urinary system is to remove waste products from your blood and help maintain the proper balance of salts and water in your body. The kidneys and ureters constitute the upper urinary tract, and the bladder and urethra make up the lower urinary tract (see Figures 2 and 3). Your kidneys filter your blood and create urine to carry away the waste. Urine is a mixture of water, salts, and urea (a waste product produced from protein metabolism). It leaves the kidneys via the ureters, the muscular tubes that deliver urine to the bladder in small amounts.

■ **The bladder.** Your bladder is the storage tank that holds urine and allows its release at the appropriate time. In the wall of this balloon-like organ is a layer of smooth muscle, called the detrusor muscle, which enables the bladder to expand and store the liquid until urination. A woman's bladder lies in front of the vagina near the uterus (where its ability to expand is noticeably lessened during pregnancy, as the uterus enlarges). A man's bladder is located below his abdomen, between the pubic bone and the rectum.

■ **The urethra.** Leading from the bladder to the outside of the body is the urethra, a slim and flexible tube surrounded by smooth muscle. At the junction where the bladder meets the urethra (called the bladder neck), two sets of muscles help hold urine in. The internal urethral sphincter is made up of involuntary muscles that keep a constant pressure on the ure-

Figure 1 Men vs. women: Urinary symptoms

URINARY PROBLEM	Women	Men
Storage problems (difficulty holding in urine, including frequency, urgency, and leakage)	59.2%	51.3%
Voiding (difficulty urinating)	19.5%	27.7%
Feeling of urgency when bladder is not full	12.8%	10.8%
Urine leakage (incontinence)	13.1%	5.4%
Stress incontinence (leakage when jumping, coughing, laughing)	6.4%	0.6%
Mixed incontinence (combination of stress and urgency)	2.4%	0.6%

Adapted from Irwin DE, et al. "Population-Based Survey of Urinary Incontinence, Overactive Bladder, and Other Lower Urinary Tract Symptoms in Five Countries: Results of the EPIC Study," European Urology (Dec. 2006).

thra without conscious effort. The external, or outer, sphincter muscles are under voluntary control. This area is also supported by collagen fibers.

In women, the urethra is only about an inch and a half long. Estrogen-sensitive cells line the urethra, producing secretions that help create a tight seal. In men, the urethra is about eight inches long, extending from between the scrotum and rectum to the tip of the penis. Near the bladder, a man's urethra passes through his prostate gland. The prostate, normally the size of a walnut, helps to support the urethra and helps with continence, but it can also create problems if it enlarges or requires removal or other surgery.

■ **Urinary support.** The urinary system, the intestines, and the reproductive organs are supported by ligaments and the pelvic floor. The pelvic floor is an important network of muscles that extends from your pubic bone to your tailbone, with openings for the urethra and anus, as well as the vagina in women. Most of the time, certain pelvic muscles stay contracted to hold the pelvic organs in place against the pull of gravity.

When you are active or trying to avoid urination, you can voluntarily tighten these muscles, along with the external urethral sphincter, to provide added support and prevent leakage. When you urinate, your pelvic floor muscles and urethral sphincter relax, and your bladder muscles contract, sending the urine from the bladder, through the urethra, and out of the body. When the bladder is empty, the bladder muscles relax, and the sphincter and pelvic muscles tighten.

■ **Urinary nerves.** The nervous system helps control urination. Before toilet training, a simple reflex controls the timing of urination. Stretch-detecting sensory nerves in the detrusor muscle signal the spinal cord that the bladder is filling with urine. In response, motor nerves from the spine signal the bladder muscles to contract and the urethra and pelvic floor mus-

Figure 2 Female urinary function

The bladder's first job is to store urine that has been filtered by the kidneys and delivered through the ureters. Once the bladder is nearly full, the nerves send a signal to the brain. To urinate, you relax the sphincter muscle, and the brain signals the bladder muscle (detrusor) to contract to push the urine out. In women, incontinence typically results from one of three main problems:

(1) the bladder's detrusor muscle can become unstable or overactive, which can cause urge and frequency incontinence;

(2) the urinary sphincter that normally opens and closes at your command may become weakened, leading to stress incontinence; or

(3) the pelvic muscles (urogenital diaphragm) may be weakened, which can also cause stress incontinence.

www.health.harvard.edu

Better Bladder and Bowel Control   3

cles to relax, allowing urination. As the brain matures, it is able to override the spinal nerves' automatic signal for the bladder to empty. The bladder gradually becomes capable of storing greater amounts of urine, and a child learns to urinate when it is convenient and socially acceptable.

Types of urinary incontinence

Many things can go wrong with the complex system that allows us to control urination. Incontinence is categorized by the type of problem and, to a lesser extent, by differences in symptoms.

Stress incontinence

If urine leaks out when you jump, cough, or laugh, you may have stress incontinence. Any physical exertion that increases abdominal pressure also puts pressure on the bladder. The word "stress" actually refers to the physical strain associated with leakage. Although it can be emotionally distressing, the condition has nothing to do with emotion. Often only a small amount of urine leaks out. In more severe cases, the pressure of a full bladder overcomes the body's ability to hold in urine. The leakage occurs even though the bladder muscles are not contracting and you don't feel the urge to urinate.

Stress incontinence occurs when the urethral sphincter, the pelvic floor muscles, or both these structures have been weakened or damaged and cannot dependably hold in urine. Stress incontinence is divided into two subtypes. In urethral hypermobility, the bladder and urethra shift downward when abdominal pressure rises, and there is no hammock-

Figure 3 Male urinary function

1. Prostate enlargement
2. Detrusor overactivity
3. Pelvic floor weakness
4. Sphincter dysfunction

The normal male bladder stores urine as it comes from the kidneys through the ureters. Once the bladder is nearly full, the nerves signal "fullness" to the brain. When you are ready, you relax your urethral sphincter, allowing the urine to flow through the urethra, past the prostate gland, and out through the penis. Incontinence can occur when prostate enlargement constricts the urethra, inhibiting the flow of urine, causing difficulty urinating and sometimes causing the bladder to overfill (1). In addition, prostate surgeries may cause damage to crucial nerves, detrusor overactivity (2), weakened pelvic floor muscles (3), or sphincter dysfunction (4).

like support for the urethra to be compressed against to keep it closed. In intrinsic sphincter deficiency, problems in the urinary sphincter interfere with full closure or allow the sphincter to pop open under pressure. Many experts believe that women who have delivered vaginally are most likely to develop stress incontinence because giving birth has stretched and possibly damaged the pelvic floor muscles and nerves (see "The childbirth connection," below). Generally, the larger the baby, the longer the labor, the older the mother, and the greater the number of births, the more likely that incontinence will result.

Age is likewise a factor in stress incontinence. As a woman gets older, the muscles in her pelvic floor and urethra weaken, and it takes less pressure for the urethra to open and allow leakage. Estrogen can also play some role, although it is not clear how much. Many women do not experience symptoms until after menopause.

In men, the most frequent cause of stress incontinence is urinary sphincter damage sustained through prostate surgery or a pelvic fracture.

Lung conditions that cause frequent coughing, such as emphysema and cystic fibrosis, can also contribute to stress incontinence in both men and women.

The childbirth connection

It's a little-known fact that many childbirth classes fail to adequately cover: an estimated 40% of women who give birth vaginally go on to develop one or more of the problems collectively known as pelvic floor disorders. These include stress incontinence, overactive bladder, uterine prolapse (in which the uterus drops out of its normal position), cystocele (in which the bladder bulges into the vagina), rectocele (in which the rectum bulges into the vagina), and fecal incontinence. These disorders often grow worse over time, requiring surgical repair in at least 11% of women over all.

Vaginal delivery can lead to pelvic floor damage as the baby stretches the pelvic floor muscles and other tissues on its way through the birth canal, sometimes causing tearing or other damage. Research results show that a number of factors raise the risk of damage for women who deliver vaginally, including these:

- older age of the mother
- greater weight of the baby
- higher number of vaginal births
- longer second stage of labor
- episiotomy (a surgical cut made to expand the vaginal opening during vaginal delivery).

What are the solutions? Delivery by cesarean section protects against severe incontinence, but some women do develop incontinence even if they have only had cesarean sections. As the rate of cesarean section continues to rise (about 31% of babies were delivered by cesarean section in 2006), many women and health professionals are concerned that too many unwarranted cesarean deliveries are performed. Research to help determine when a cesarean is the best choice is ongoing.

Women with some of the above risk factors should bear them in mind when considering their birth options. Researchers who published a study in the journal *Obstetrics and Gynecology* in 2006 suggested that health professionals inform their patients that cesarean delivery would reduce the risk of pelvic floor injury by 85%. This study of 4,458 women found that stress incontinence was 86% more likely in women who delivered vaginally compared with those who had cesarean section. Anal incontinence was 72% more common, and overactive bladder was 53% more common. But even cesarean delivery can, in rare cases, cause incontinence, and because cesarean delivery comes with its own set of risks, each woman should discuss her situation thoroughly with her obstetrician while making plans for childbirth.

The use of episiotomy during childbirth has declined steadily, but millions of women have had episiotomy in the past. It was previously believed that episiotomy helped prevent tearing of the vagina and damage to the pelvic floor. However, evidence has failed to confirm any benefit. And episiotomy may cause more damage than it prevents. For example, a 2006 study in *Obstetrics and Gynecology* found that women who had episiotomy were the most likely to experience tears in the anal sphincter. After sphincter tear and repair, about half of women experience fecal or gas incontinence. For many women, the symptoms improve or disappear within a few months, but others sustain persistent or worsening problems, or find that symptoms reappear after subsequent deliveries. Besides episiotomy, other major factors contributing to sphincter tears were heavier babies, a prolonged second stage of labor, and forceps delivery. Vacuum delivery did not lead to sphincter tear. Gentle delivery techniques and slow, gradual induction (when induction is necessary) would go a long way toward sparing women incontinence resulting from childbirth.

Pregnant women can talk with their health care providers in advance about their specific risk factors for pelvic damage and consider their childbirth choices in the context of these risk factors. Women who already have symptoms of pelvic floor damage can learn more about treatment options in this report.

> ### Key-in-the-door syndrome
>
> Do you get an overwhelming urge to urinate just when you arrive home and start to open the door? Also called "latch-key incontinence," this phenomenon is a good demonstration of the bladder-brain connection. When you feel the urge to urinate as you're going home, you suppress it until you arrive. Eventually, the bladder becomes conditioned to associate arriving home with urinating, and the urge comes on whether or not your bladder is full. This is not a "psychological" problem, but a reflex-conditioning problem, much as when you salivate upon smelling something good to eat.

Overactive bladder (urge incontinence)

If you feel a strong urge to urinate even when your bladder isn't full, your incontinence might be related to overactive bladder, sometimes called urge incontinence. This condition occurs in both men and women and involves an overwhelming urge to urinate immediately, frequently followed by loss of urine before you can reach a bathroom (see "Key-in-the-door syndrome," above). Even if you never have an accident, urgency and urinary frequency can interfere with work and a social life because of the need to keep running to the bathroom.

Urgency is caused when the bladder muscle, the detrusor, begins to contract and signals a need to urinate, even when the bladder is not full. Another name for this phenomenon is detrusor overactivity.

Overactive bladder can result from physical problems that keep your body from halting involuntary bladder muscle contractions. Such problems include damage to the brain, the spine, or the nerves extending from the spine to the bladder—for example, from an accident, diabetes, or neurological disease. Irritating substances within the bladder, such as those produced during an infection, might also cause the bladder muscle to contract.

Often there is no identifiable cause for overactive bladder, but people are more likely to develop the problem as they age. Postmenopausal women, in particular, tend to develop this condition, perhaps because of age-related changes in the bladder lining and muscle. African American women with incontinence are more likely to report symptoms of overactive bladder than stress incontinence, while the reverse is true in white women.

A condition called myofascial pelvic pain syndrome has been identified with symptoms that include overactive bladder accompanied by pain in the pelvic area or a sense of aching, heaviness, or burning.

In addition, infections of the urinary tract, bladder, or prostate can cause temporary urgency. Partial blockage of the urinary tract by a bladder stone, a tumor (rarely), or, in men, an enlarged prostate (a condition known as benign prostatic hyperplasia, or BPH) can cause urgency, frequency, and sometimes urge incontinence. Surgery for prostate cancer or BPH can trigger symptoms of overactive bladder, as can freezing (cryotherapy) and radiation seed treatment (brachytherapy) for prostate cancer.

Neurological diseases (such as Parkinson's disease and multiple sclerosis) can also result in urge incontinence, as can a stroke. When hospitalized following a stroke, 40% to 60% of patients have incontinence; by the time they are discharged, 25% still have it, and one year later, 15% do.

Mixed incontinence

If you have symptoms of both overactive bladder and stress incontinence, you likely have mixed incontinence, a combination of both types. Most women with incontinence have both stress and urge symptoms—a challenging situation. Mixed incontinence also occurs in men who have had prostate removal or surgery for an enlarged prostate, and in frail older people of either sex.

Overflow incontinence

If your bladder never completely empties, you might experience urine leakage, with or without feeling a need to go. Overflow incontinence occurs when something blocks urine from flowing normally out of the bladder, as in the case of prostate enlargement that partially closes off the urethra. It can also occur in both men and women if the bladder muscle becomes underactive (the opposite of an overactive bladder) so you don't feel an urge to urinate. Eventually the bladder becomes overfilled, or distended, pulling the urethra open and allowing urine to leak out. The bladder might also spasm at random times, causing leakage. This condition is sometimes related to diabetes or cardiovascular disease.

Men are much more frequently diagnosed with overflow incontinence than women because it is often caused by prostate-related conditions. In addition to enlarged prostate, other possible causes of urine blockage include tumors, bladder stones, or scar tissue. If a woman has severe prolapse of her uterus or bladder (meaning that the organ has dropped out of its proper position), her urethra can become kinked like a bent garden hose, interfering with the flow of urine.

Nerve damage (from injuries, childbirth, past surgeries, or diseases such as diabetes, multiple sclerosis, or shingles) and aging often prevent the bladder muscle from contracting normally. Medications that prevent bladder muscle contraction or that make you unaware of the urge to urinate can also result in overflow incontinence.

Functional incontinence

If your urinary tract is functioning properly but other illnesses or disabilities are preventing you from staying dry, you might have what is known as functional incontinence.

For example, if an illness rendered you unaware or unconcerned about the need to find a toilet, you would become incontinent. Medications, dementia, or mental illness can decrease awareness of the need to find a toilet.

Even if your urinary system is fine, it can be extremely difficult for you to avoid accidents if you have trouble getting to a toilet. This problem can affect anyone with a condition that makes it excessively difficult to move to the bathroom and undress in time. This includes problems as diverse as having arthritis, being hospitalized or restrained, or having a toilet located too far away.

If a medication (such as a diuretic used to treat high blood pressure or heart failure) causes you to produce abnormally large amounts of urine, you could develop incontinence that requires a change in treatment. If you make most of your urine at night, the result might be nocturnal incontinence, or bedwetting.

Reflex incontinence

Reflex incontinence occurs when the bladder muscle contracts and urine leaks (often in large amounts) without any warning or urge. This can happen as a result of damage to the nerves that normally warn the brain that the bladder is filling. Reflex incontinence usually appears in people with serious neurological impairment from multiple sclerosis, spinal cord injury, other injuries, or damage from surgery or radiation treatment.

Table 1 Medications that can cause urinary incontinence

MEDICATION	EFFECT	SYMPTOMS
Diuretics, such as hydrochlorothiazide (Esidrix, Hydrodiuril, Oretic), furosemide (Lasix), bumetanide (Bumex), triamterene with hydrochlorothiazide (Maxzide)	Increase urine production by the kidney.	Frequent urination, overactive bladder, stress incontinence.
Muscle relaxants and sedatives, such as diazepam (Valium), chlordiazepoxide (Librium), lorazepam (Ativan)	Cause sedation or drowsiness, relax urethra.	Frequent urination, stress incontinence, lack of concern or desire to use the toilet.
Narcotics, such as oxycodone (Percocet), meperidine (Demerol), morphine	Cause sedation or drowsiness; relax bladder, causing retention of urine.	Lack of concern or desire to use the toilet, difficulty in starting urinary stream, straining to void, voiding with a weak stream, leaking between urinations, frequency incontinence.
Antihistamines, such as diphenhydramine (Benadryl) Anticholinergics and calcium-channel blockers, such as verapamil (Calan), nifedipine (Procardia), diltiazem (Cardizem)	Relax bladder, causing retention of urine; in some cases, increase urine production.	Difficulty in starting the urinary stream, straining to void, voiding with a weak stream, leaking between urinations.
Alpha-adrenergic antagonists, such as terazosin (Hytrin), doxazosin (Cardura)	Relax the bladder outlet muscle.	Leaking when coughing, sneezing, laughing, exercising, etc.

Evaluating urinary incontinence

Many people never tell a physician that they are incontinent, and that leads to prolonged and largely needless suffering. In 70% of cases, incontinence can be cured or significantly improved. The treatment of incontinence has advanced greatly and is changing all the time, so don't be reluctant to seek help now, even if previous attempts brought little relief.

Depending on the complexity of your symptoms, you can choose to visit your primary care physician or go to a specialist (see "Choosing a clinician," page 22). If you are comfortable with your primary care physician, start there. If your symptoms seem to be connected with a specific medical event, such as childbirth, surgery, or starting a new prescription, the physician involved in that treatment might be your first choice. A woman may choose to see a urogynecologist—a gynecologist with board-certified special training and an interest in incontinence. A man who has had prostate symptoms or treatment may choose to consult a urologist. Physicians vary widely in their training and interest in incontinence. If a physician seems uncomfortable or uninformed discussing the subject, presents limited options, or seems unduly pessimistic about your condition, seek another opinion.

To pinpoint and treat the underlying problem, your physician will need you to describe your symptoms in as much detail as possible. You might be asked to keep a diary of urinations and fluid intake for a few days (see "Keeping a bladder diary," page 16). At your visit, be prepared to give a full medical history, including details on all surgeries, pregnancies, and any medications you are taking (see Table 1). You may also need to answer specific questions such as these:

- When did the incontinence start?
- How often do you have leakage?

▶ Is it cancer?

Incontinence can be a symptom of bladder cancer, but it is rarely the first or only sign of this disease. If you have other symptoms, such as blood in your urine, your physician is likely to suggest specific tests to rule out bladder cancer. Bladder cancer is much less common than cancers of the colon, lungs, breast, or prostate.

- Is it worse during the day or night?
- What brings it on? Do you have any warning?
- What makes it worse?
- Does anything make it better?
- Do you generally leak a little (damp underwear), a moderate amount (your underwear is soaked), or a lot (your clothing gets soaked and all the urine in your bladder comes out)?
- Do you leak urine during intercourse or with orgasm?
- What is your typical fluid intake (including caffeinated and alcoholic beverages)?
- How often do you go to the toilet to empty your bladder during the daytime? How often when you are trying to sleep?
- Do you have other problems urinating? After you urinate, does your bladder still feel full? Do you have trouble starting the urine flow? Is the stream weak or strong? Is urination ever painful?
- Have you also had trouble controlling your bowel movements?
- Are you using pads or other means to manage your incontinence? How is it working? Have you altered your activities because of incontinence?

The physical exam

For this exam, your clinician places more focus on your nervous system, abdomen, and genital area than during a standard physical. The clinician checks your reflexes, assesses your muscle strength, and observes whether you can distinguish the touch of something sharp from something dull. To test nerves in the genital area, the doctor may stroke the skin near your anus and watch for a normal muscle contraction. In women, the doctor gently taps the clitoris and looks for a subtle muscle contraction of the anus, which is a normal reflex.

None of these tests is painful or uncomfortable. If the doctor observes problems with any functions that rely on the same nerves as those that control urinary continence, it can mean that these nerves are involved in your bladder symptoms.

During the abdominal exam, the doctor presses on your abdomen to feel your bladder and check other areas for hernias, tenderness, or any signs of tumor, infection, scarring from previous surgeries, or an impacted bowel.

Both men and women provide a urine sample, which is checked immediately for blood, sugar, or large amounts of bacteria (normal urine is sterile). Blood can indicate irritation of the urinary tract. If there is such irritation, the cause must be determined. If sugar is detected, your physician might suspect diabetes, which can increase your urine volume and make incontinence more likely. Bacteria indicate possible infection. As a more specific test, a urine sample may be sent to a laboratory to be cultured; if harmful bacteria are detected, a sensitivity test can identify the appropriate antibiotic to treat the infection.

■ **For women.** During a thorough pelvic exam, the clinician inserts a gloved finger into the vagina to help assess the strength of the pelvic floor muscles and to see whether the bladder or uterus has prolapsed (dropped out of normal position). If you hear the word "POP" it may mean your clinician is using the Pelvic Organ Prolapse Quantification system, also called the "POP-Q" system, as a way of measuring and grading the degree of prolapse of the pelvic organs to help guide decisions about treatment.

The clinician might ask you to contract your muscles as if you were trying to avoid urinating or passing gas, or to cough during the exam to see if urine spurts out of the urethra. The clinician might repeat the exam while you are in a standing position.

With a speculum in place, the clinician observes whether the tissue lining your vagina shows atrophy or other signs that it lacks estrogen. That would indicate that your urethral lining (not visible during the exam) is likely to show a similar lack of this hormone. The clinician may insert a Q-tip coated with numbing jelly (such as Xylocaine) into your urethra just up into the bladder to observe how the angle of the Q-tip changes when you bear down as if trying to have a bowel movement. A large change indicates poor support of the urethra and points toward a diagnosis of stress incontinence.

The clinician might also look for direct evidence of stress incontinence. You may be asked to stand with one leg up on a stool, holding a paper towel over your crotch; if urine appears on the paper towel after you cough, that's a positive stress test. This test is usually performed at the beginning of your physical, when you have a full bladder. Afterward, you can urinate to increase your comfort during the rest of the exam.

Occasionally, if stress incontinence is suspected but is not observed during the exam, the clinician may give you a pre-weighed pad to wear while doing a series of exercises. The pad is then weighed again to determine how much leakage has occurred. You might go home with a package of pads to wear and save in sealed plastic bags over a 24-hour period, so that total leakage can be estimated.

■ **For men.** The doctor examines the penis for signs of constriction of the foreskin or an abnormal narrowing, or stenosis, of the urethra, which can result from scarring or infection. The doctor conducts a digital rectal exam, which involves inserting a gloved finger into the rectum to feel the size and texture of the prostate gland and assess the strength of the pelvic muscles. You may be asked to contract your muscles as if you were trying to avoid urinating or passing gas.

SPECIAL SECTION

Urodynamic testing

If your condition is not easily diagnosed by a physical exam and a discussion of your symptoms, or if previous treatments have not improved your symptoms of incontinence, your doctor may suggest urodynamic testing, a series of specialized tests that help evaluate your urinary system in action. Many doctors who diagnose patients with urinary problems have a urodynamic testing lab outfitted with a special chair and computer equipment that can help obtain measurements of urinary pressure and flow.

Urodynamic testing is available for both men and women. For women, the testing may be done by a physician who is a urogynecologist, a doctor certified in this board-certified subspecialty. A technician in the doctor's office may also perform the testing. Men should consult a urologist, another board-certified specialist.

The usefulness of urodynamic testing depends on the experience of the tester, the choice of tests, and the type of incontinence. For example, urodynamic tests are very sensitive in detecting stress incontinence, but asking patients about their symptoms is almost as good, and is even more effective when supplemented with a bladder diary.

Urodynamic testing will likely be recommended if your symptoms point toward more than one type of incontinence, if you have had previous surgery on your bladder or sphincters, if surgery is planned, or if you do not improve after standard treatments.

Your urodynamic test is likely to include one or more of the following procedures.

Uroflowmetry

For this test, you start with a full bladder and urinate into a funnel at a special urinal or commode that automatically measures the amount you produce and the rate of the flow. A slow flow might

Figure 4 Detecting bladder problems

Photo courtesy of May M. Wakamatsu, M.D.

Before you begin urodynamic testing, your doctor will ask you to describe your symptoms and your personal health history. Once you are in the urodynamic testing lab (above), you'll sit in a specially designed chair equipped with sensitive catheters that feed information from your bladder to a computer that records bladder volume, pressure, rate of flow, and leakage.

Urodynamic testing | SPECIAL SECTION

indicate an obstruction in the urethra or a weak bladder muscle. This test is quick and noninvasive.

Post-void residual volume

This test measures the amount of urine left in your bladder after you urinate. Two techniques are used to measure this. The physician may insert a flexible tube (called a catheter) through your urethra into the bladder to draw off the remaining fluid (which also provides an uncontaminated sample for urine culture and prepares you for further tests). Being catheterized usually causes only mild discomfort. Alternatively, the amount of urine in your bladder can be visualized using a specialized ultrasound machine called a bladder scanner. This is quicker and more comfortable, and it avoids the possibility that inserting a catheter could cause an infection or traumatize the lining of the urethra. However, it can be less accurate.

Measuring residual urine volume is particularly valuable if you are troubled by repeated urinary tract infections, if you have a neurological disorder, or if your doctor suspects that a blockage is preventing your bladder from emptying properly.

Cystometry

This test monitors how the pressure builds up in your bladder as it fills with urine, how much urine your bladder can hold, and at what point you feel the urge to urinate (see Figure 5).

During cystometry, a very narrow catheter is placed in your bladder to measure pressure. Through the catheter, the technician slowly fills your bladder with sterile water. The catheter measures the pressure inside your bladder and can measure the pressure inside the urethra; an additional small pressure catheter may also be inserted into your rectum (for men) or vagi-

Figure 5 Pressure test (Cystometry)

For men or women, a cystometry test measures the pressure in the bladder, urethra, and abdomen. A catheter in the bladder fills the bladder with fluid and measures pressure in centimeters of water. Another catheter, placed in the vagina for women or the rectum for men, reflects the pressure in the abdomen. Cystometry can reveal detrusor overactivity, stress incontinence from sphincter weakness, or weak pelvic floor muscles.

www.health.harvard.edu

Better Bladder and Bowel Control

SPECIAL SECTION | **Urodynamic testing**

nal canal (for women). You tell the physician when you first feel the urge to urinate, when the urge becomes strong, and other sensations (pain, temperature changes, and the symptoms that brought you to the doctor).

This test detects abnormal contractions or spasms of your detrusor muscle during filling, indicating incontinence caused by an overactive bladder (either alone or along with stress incontinence). At several points during the filling, you may be asked to cough or bear down so the doctor can see whether fluid comes out of the urethra. This measurement is sometimes called leak point pressure.

A low leak point pressure is a sign of stress incontinence. If it is extremely low (you start to leak as soon as you begin bearing down), it may mean that age-related changes or scar tissue is preventing your urethra from closing well enough to prevent urine leakage, resulting in the type of stress incontinence called intrinsic sphincter deficiency.

Once your bladder is filled to the point where you have a strong urge, you will urinate, and the pressure and volume are measured. By monitoring pressure while you urinate, this test can distinguish whether a low flow is due to weak bladder contractions or something blocking the flow. Portions of the test may be repeated while you are in a standing position, which makes stress incontinence more apparent.

In women, urogynecologists often perform a test called a urethral pressure profile. The bladder/urethral catheter is drawn through the urethra very slowly, and the urethral pressure is measured. If the pressure is low, that indicates your urethral sphincter is weak, which causes stress incontinence.

Electromyography (EMG)

In this test, small electrode patches are placed in the crotch area to pick up electrical current that is created when the pelvic floor muscles contract. Called a surface EMG, this test may help determine whether the activities of the bladder and urethra are coordinated with each other.

If your doctor suspects that the nerves to your urinary sphincter are seriously damaged, or that the sphincter muscle is responding inappropriately to nerve signals, he or she may insert a thin needle electrode into the muscle of the urethra to perform a more accurate EMG. This test may also be performed by a neurologist. Because most people find the EMG causes some pain, it is not done routinely.

Cystography

A cystogram, or voiding cystourethrogram, is an x-ray test. The test itself may be performed during cystometry or uroflowmetry, or both, but a fluid visible on x-ray is substituted for the sterile water. At various points in the process, x-rays are taken as you cough or bear down and as you urinate. This test can pinpoint the location of a blockage or reveal an abnormally open urethra.

Video-urodynamic study

Using highly specialized equipment, this technique combines cystometry, uroflowmetry, and cystography into a single computerized test. This equipment can simultaneously measure urine flow and pressure in the bladder and rectum. The test may provide useful information about your bladder and urethral func-

---

After urodynamic testing

You might have mild discomfort or soreness for a few hours after these tests. Drinking two large glasses of water each hour for two hours may help ease your symptoms. Ask your doctor whether you can take a warm bath. If not, you may be able to hold a warm, damp washcloth over the urethral opening to relieve the discomfort. Your doctor may give you an antibiotic to take for one to two days to prevent an infection. If you have signs of infection, fever, chills, or pain, call your doctor.

Results: For some of the more simple tests, you may get answers as the test is being done or right after it's done. For others, it will take a few days.

tion, especially if you have problems voiding (such as being able to begin urinating only in a certain position). The equipment for video-urodynamic testing is expensive and not widely used.

Other evaluation procedures

Depending on your symptoms, other tests may be performed at the same visit as your urodynamic testing.

Cystoscopy

Using a lighted telescope at the end of a thin tube called a cystoscope, your doctor can inspect the inside of your urethra and bladder for signs of infection, abnormal growths, bladder stones, scarring, or improperly placed stitches from previous surgeries. This test is used in both men and women, but it is easier for women to undergo comfortably because the urethra is shorter.

For the test, you lie on your back. A numbing jelly is placed into your urethra, and the cystoscope is inserted until the end is inside your bladder. Sterile water is passed through the thin tube to fill your bladder and optimize the picture. You may feel some discomfort and the need to urinate when your bladder is filled. After about three to five minutes, the cystoscope is removed, and you can use the toilet.

Ultrasound

Ultrasound uses sound waves rather than x-rays to create an image of internal organs. You may undergo an abdominal or transvaginal ultrasound exam to look at the structure and position of your kidneys, bladder, and prostate; to visualize leakage in stress incontinence; to detect abnormalities such as tumors, kidney stones, or fibroids; or to evaluate treatment with bulking agents (see "Injection of bulking agents," page 24). An ultrasound exam takes about half an hour and is painless.

Intravenous pyelogram or urogram

This test creates a picture of your kidneys and ureters. A dye is injected into your bloodstream through your arm. The dye is excreted through the kidneys and collects in urine, allowing an x-ray to reveal the structure of the kidneys and ureters and any areas where fluid may be escaping or is blocked.

Treating urinary incontinence

Treatment choices for urinary incontinence range from lifestyle changes to surgery. Your treatment will depend on the underlying problems causing the incontinence. But keep in mind that no treatment works perfectly, and you may have to try more than one approach before you find the one that best suits your needs (see "What to do for urinary incontinence," below). Treatments may be different for men and women. Because there are a variety of options, your preferences are important in developing a plan.

It's also important to know that less invasive treatments, such as biofeedback or pelvic floor exercises, are a good first step and can be helpful, but may not be as effective as some surgical procedures. Even surgical treatments are becoming less invasive and requiring shorter recovery times. You and your physician need to decide which is most appropriate for you. Check with your health plan to find out which therapies are covered. Treatment for urinary incontinence is an area of active research, and new approaches are under development.

Bladder training

You might be teaching your bladder some bad habits—habits that can gradually result in incontinence or frequent bathroom breaks. For example, if you routinely urinate before your bladder is full, the bladder learns to signal the need to go when less volume is present. That can set up a vicious cycle, as you respond to the new urges and teach your bladder to cry "run" when less and less urine is present.

Luckily, old bladders can learn new tricks. Bladder training, a program of urinating on schedule, enables you to gradually increase the amount of urine you can comfortably hold. Bladder training is a mainstay of

---

Quick Guide: What to do for urinary incontinence

Lifestyle changes
- Bladder training (overactive bladder)
- Fluid management (overactive bladder and stress incontinence)
- Pelvic floor physical therapy (overactive bladder and stress incontinence)
- Biofeedback (overactive bladder and stress incontinence)

Muscle conditioning without exercise
- Electrical stimulation (overactive bladder and stress incontinence)

Medications
- Alpha-adrenergic agonists (stress incontinence)
- Anticholinergics (overactive bladder)
- Cholinergics (overflow incontinence)
- DDAVP (bedwetting)
- Tricyclic antidepressants (overactive bladder and nocturia)
- Alpha-adrenergic antagonists (for men, for overflow incontinence)
- Estrogen (for women, for overactive bladder and stress incontinence; evidence of efficacy is inconclusive)

Surgical procedures
- Sling, male and female versions (stress incontinence)
- Bladder neck suspension, Burch procedure, open or laparoscopic (stress incontinence)
- Artificial urinary sphincter (reflex and stress incontinence); rarely used in women
- Sacral neuromodulation (severe overactive bladder in men; overflow incontinence; incontinence related to overactive bladder, urinary retention, or frequency in women)

Other procedures
- Injection of bulking agents (stress incontinence)
- Percutaneous tibial nerve stimulation (overactive bladder)
- Injection of botulinum toxin (overactive bladder)

treatment for urinary frequency and overactive bladder in both women and men, alone or in conjunction with medications or other techniques. It can also help prevent or lessen symptoms of overactive bladder that may emerge after surgery for stress incontinence.

In one study, women ages 55 and older who participated in six weekly bladder training sessions had half as many episodes of leakage compared with a group of women who didn't undergo bladder training.

You can see a health professional for bladder training, or you can try bladder training on your own. Because bladder training is low-cost and low-risk, your clinician may encourage you to try it first, even before specific diagnostic tests are performed. Here's a step-by-step bladder-training technique:

- **Keep track.** For a day or two, keep track of the times you urinate or leak urine during the day (see "Keeping a bladder diary," page 16).
- **Calculate.** On average, how many hours do you wait between urinations during the day?
- **Choose an interval.** Based on your typical interval between urinations, select a starting interval for training that is 15 minutes longer. If your typical interval is one hour, make your starting interval one hour and 15 minutes.
- **Hold back.** When you start training, empty your bladder first thing in the morning and not again until the interval you've set. If the time arrives before you feel the urge, go anyway. If the urge hits first, remind yourself that your bladder isn't really full, and use whatever techniques you can to delay going. Try the pelvic floor exercises sometimes called Kegels (see "Pelvic floor exercises," page 16), or simply try to wait another five minutes before walking slowly to the bathroom.
- **Increase your interval.** Once you are comfortable with your set interval, increase it by 15 minutes. Over several weeks or months, you may find you are able to wait much longer and that you experience far fewer feelings of urgency or episodes of urge incontinence. After four to eight weeks, if you think you have improved, do another diary. Compare your initial diary to your second diary to note the improvements in voiding intervals and voided volumes—this process reinforces the bladder training process.

Fluid management

Do you have a drinking problem? Not just alcohol, but water, soda, coffee, tea, or juice? For some people, eliminating excess fluid intake is all it takes to bring incontinence under control. For example, in a British study, reducing fluid intake by 25%—enjoying your usual beverages, but pouring each cup or glass only three-quarters full—significantly reduced overactive bladder symptoms and nocturia. Or you can use the following fluid-management technique along with your bladder-training program or other treatments.

Review your bladder diary (see page 16) to see how much fluid you're drinking each day. Once your physician reviews this information, he or she may suggest changes in the amount of fluid you consume. If your urine output is much higher than 48 ounces, you may be drinking too much fluid. This isn't necessarily unhealthy, but it forces your bladder to handle more urine and may invite or aggravate incontinence. Cutting back may be helpful.

On the other hand, if your output is much lower than 30 to 40 ounces, it can increase your risk for urinary tract infection and, in some people, create a frequent urge to urinate because the concentrated urine irritates the bladder lining. Unless you engage in strenuous exercise or have a medical condition (such as a propensity toward forming kidney stones) that requires more fluid consumption, you can try these guidelines to improve your symptoms:

- Watch your fluid intake. Drink only when you feel thirsty, and don't exceed six to eight 8-ounce cups of fluid per day from all sources, including soup or milk in your cereal, unless you have a medical condition that requires more. Note that an 8-ounce cup is only two-thirds of a standard soda can.

- Don't drink more than 8 ounces at a time.

- Don't guzzle. The faster your bladder fills, the more likely you are to feel urgency.

- Minimize caffeinated and carbonated drinks.

- Decrease or eliminate alcohol consumption.

- If you are thirsty because it is hot or you have exercised, don't hesitate to drink water.

Pelvic floor exercises

Another approach for men and women who want to try nonsurgical methods first is to strengthen the muscles of the pelvic floor through exercise. The strength and proper action of your pelvic floor muscles are important in maintaining continence. Like weakened or damaged muscles elsewhere in your body, their condition can usually be improved with regular exercise and, if needed, physical therapy.

It may seem odd, but tight pelvic floor muscles, too, can cause incontinence. That's because tight muscles (resulting from pelvic, back, or hip surgery or other causes) can't relax when they are supposed to. And when the time comes for them to contract to control the flow of urine, they can't because they are already tightly contracted. Instead, they go into spasm. This condition is often best treated by pelvic floor physical therapy performed by a qualified pelvic floor physical therapist.

Basic pelvic muscle exercises are often called Kegel exercises, named for Arnold Kegel, the physician who first developed them. Regular Kegel exercises may be helpful particularly for women with mild to moderate stress incontinence. Learning to perform a strong and fast pelvic muscle contraction just before and during actions that commonly cause problems for those with stress incontinence (such as coughing or jumping) reduces leakage. Pelvic muscle exercises may help overactive bladder and mixed incontinence as well.

For men, Kegels can help prevent post-void dribbling (see "Dribble relief," page 31). But studies have not shown Kegel exercises alone to be particularly effective in preventing or treating incontinence that results from prostate surgery.

Because Kegels cost nothing and are quite safe, they are recommended for most patients, either alone or in combination with other treatments. To perform

Keeping a bladder diary

Complete the information for two consecutive 24-hour periods. Record both day and night.
- Begin with first urination upon arising.
- Record intake amount in ounces and type of fluid (for example, coffee, juice, water, etc.).
- Record approximate urine output and time of urination.

	FLUID INTAKE		FLUID OUTPUT		
	Time of intake (a.m./p.m.)	Amount and type of fluid (oz)	Time of void (a.m./p.m.)	Amount voided (oz)	Leakage (time, place, quantity)
Day 1					
Day 2					

a Kegel, you first need to find your pelvic floor muscles and then repeatedly contract and relax them.

- **Locate your pelvic muscles.** Pretend you are trying to avoid passing gas; if you are a woman, you can pretend to tighten your vagina around a tampon. Both actions involve the pelvic muscles. You will feel a correct contraction more in the back than the front, like you are pulling the anal area in or stopping gas from escaping.
- **Choose your position.** You can start by lying on your back until you get the feel of contracting the pelvic floor muscles. Later, you can practice while sitting and standing as well.
- **Practice contractions.** Practice both short contractions and releases (sometimes called "quick flicks") and longer ones (gradually increasing the strength of the contraction and holding it at your maximum for up to 10 seconds). Consciously relax the muscles between each repetition, and hold the relaxation phase for the same amount of time as the contraction.
- **Keep other muscles relaxed.** When doing pelvic floor exercises, don't push out your abdominal muscles, contract your leg or buttock muscles, or lift your pelvis. Place a hand gently on your belly to detect unwanted abdominal action.
- **Repetitions.** Your health professional may advise you how many Kegel exercises to do. It is more effective to spread the exercises throughout the day than to do them all at once. One simple starting regimen is to do 10 before getting out of bed, 10 standing after lunch, 10 in the evening while sitting watching TV, and another 10 before going to sleep. You can do them at other times as well: in the car sitting at a stoplight, waiting for an elevator, or waiting in a grocery line.
- **Determine your strategy.** You can practice using these exercises to control your symptoms. If you have stress incontinence, tighten your pelvic floor muscles just before lifting, coughing, laughing, or whatever usually causes urine leakage. Do the same several times when you have the urge to urinate and doubt you are going to make it to the toilet. This should relax your bladder muscle so you can walk to the toilet under control.
- **Be consistent.** Practice consistently, using whatever schedule works for you. It may take a few months for you to notice an improvement in your symptoms.

Pelvic floor physical therapy

Your physician may recommend seeing a physical therapist with training in pelvic floor therapy. Many people find it useful to have a trained expert help them identify the proper muscles and teach them to perform exercises correctly. A physical therapist trained in this specialty can also use biofeedback to aid in the process or electrical stimulation (see page 19) to help strengthen weak muscles.

Body posture, also known as body mechanics, is another important part of keeping pelvic floor muscles and structures functioning as they should be. In addition, a physical therapist with specialty training can advise a patient on bladder training and lifestyle modifications and can provide regular reinforcement and advice.

Not all physical therapists have expertise in bladder training, so ask about it before you begin your physical therapy sessions.

Using biofeedback to learn pelvic floor exercises

Both men and women can make use of biofeedback, a technique that uses a device to detect information about a biological function (for example, heart rate, skin temperature, or muscle tension) and provides feedback so you can gain greater awareness and control over that function. Biofeedback is performed by a trained practitioner such as a licensed physical therapist (see above). Home biofeedback units are also available (see page 18).

In the case of incontinence, biofeedback can help you identify pelvic floor muscles and learn to strengthen and control them in order to lessen stress incontinence, overactive bladder, and mixed incontinence.

For a biofeedback session, the practitioner inserts a small monitor into your vagina or rectum, or both. Electrodes may also be pasted on your belly to monitor abdominal contractions. As you perform your assigned pelvic exercises, you watch a computer screen and see a line or image (such as clouds or birds) rising as you contract the correct muscles more strongly. Some people have a single training session using biofeedback, while others go for six or more sessions spread over several weeks.

Some devices are available to help you do pelvic muscle exercises consistently and effectively at home. Research shows that vaginal weighted cones and home biofeedback devices yield comparable results to pelvic floor exercises. Be aware that many pieces of equipment sold via the Internet for urinary incontinence have not been tested for effectiveness. For example, exercise contraptions that you squeeze between your legs generally do not work because they don't exercise the right muscles.

■ **Vaginal weighted cones.** Some women find that using vaginal weighted cones helps boost the power of their pelvic floor exercises. These are a set of smooth, tampon-shaped inserts of increasing weight. If you have significant uterine prolapse or a rectocele, your doctor will probably not recommend this method for strengthening your pelvic muscles.

To use vaginal cones, start with the lightest (less than one ounce) and insert the cone into your vagina as you would a tampon. A lubricant may make insertion more comfortable, but it also makes the cones slippery. Then, contract your pelvic muscles to hold it in place. If contracting your muscles pushes the cone out, it may not be inserted far enough, or you may be pushing out with your abdominal muscles.

Vaginal cones function both as a strengthening tool and as a simple biofeedback device. If the cone stays in, you're contracting your muscles correctly. Start with three to five minutes, twice a day. Work up to 15 minutes, twice a day. Once you can hold a cone in place while walking, coughing, or going up and down stairs, switch to the next heavier cone.

■ **Home biofeedback devices.** These handheld electronic devices let you know how strongly you are contracting your pelvic muscles when you practice Kegels. Muscle strength is detected with a vaginal sensor and displayed on the handheld component. FDA-approved systems (such as Myself or the PFX Pelvic Floor Exerciser) are available without a prescription. In other systems, you buy the vaginal probe and rent the biofeedback device by the month. The PFX device is available in a men's model that uses an anal probe.

▶ **How much should you drink?**

The old advice to drink at least eight cups of water a day no longer holds water, particularly if you are prone to urinary incontinence.

Where did this recommendation come from? Some experts think it was based on a misunderstanding. It has been traced to the 1940s, when the National Academy of Sciences published a recommended daily allowance of 1 milliliter of fluid for each calorie burned—a little over eight cups for a typical 2,000-calorie diet. However, the statement then explained that most of this fluid could be obtained via the liquid contained in foods.

Regardless, the eight-glasses-a-day dictum caught on. Indeed, today people frequently consume much more as they tote giant water bottles, buy super-sized soft drinks, and follow the dictates of programs that promise you can lose weight by drinking as much as a quart of fluid at a time. Other people drink extra water or other liquids as part of a special diet that purports to purify or detoxify the liver or other body organs.

In a 2000 survey conducted for Rockefeller University and the International Bottled Water Association, 2,818 adults in 14 cities reported drinking about six cups of water a day—a result that was presented as alarming evidence that Americans were becoming dehydrated. But if you include the sodas, coffee, tea, milk, juice, sports drinks, and alcoholic beverages these respondents drank, their average fluid consumption was 17.6 cups a day—enough to have you urinate every waking hour, even if you don't have any problem with bladder capacity.

A kidney specialist at Dartmouth Medical School searched the scientific literature for studies that might support the idea that people need eight glasses of fluid a day. Not only did he determine that no such evidence exists, but he concluded that the research that has been done "strongly suggests that such large amounts are not needed."

Additionally, the concept of detoxifying the liver or other organs by drinking extra water or other liquids is not based on fact. A person with normal liver and kidney function can rest assured that these organs will rid the body of toxins as part of their normal function. And drinking water won't help you lose weight unless you are drinking it to replace high-calorie drinks you might ordinarily consume, such as soda and fruit juice.

Electrical stimulation

Some men and women find that they are unable to exercise their pelvic muscles consistently or effectively, or would appreciate help in beginning to condition the muscles. Often called "electro-stim," this method can be used to strengthen muscles to improve stress incontinence or to help relax muscles to improve overactive bladder.

Men and women can use either a portable device at home (such as Liberty, by Utah Medical) or a larger system in a health professional's office. A small electrode, placed inside a woman's vagina or a man's or woman's rectum, delivers an electrical current that can spur your pelvic muscles to contract painlessly. You will feel as though you are doing a Kegel. The instruments can be set for different strengths of stimulation and various time intervals of contraction and relaxation.

For stress incontinence, electrical stimulation is believed to work by strengthening the muscle. For overactive bladder, a different frequency may help reset your nervous system's control over the bladder muscle. Medicare will cover pelvic muscle stimulation if it is prescribed by your physician and you can document that you have tried standard pelvic muscle exercises for four weeks and not gotten relief.

Medication to treat urinary incontinence

Although there are no medications designed specifically to treat stress incontinence, certain drugs occasionally help with the symptoms, and others are useful for both urge and stress symptoms (see Table 2). In men who have overflow incontinence caused by an enlarged prostate, medications to shrink the prostate may help. Patients and clinicians can work together to find the medication that results in the fewest side effects, at the lowest dose that eases symptoms. This may take some trial and error.

Before starting any new medication, inform your doctor about any other drugs you are taking. Some medications may be unsafe or ineffective when combined with an incontinence medication. Before prescribing a medication for incontinence, your doctor will also want to make certain that no other drug you are taking could be causing your incontinence (see Table 1). If so, changing that prescription might solve the problem without introducing a new medication.

Along with medication, your doctor may suggest you use Kegel exercises to improve the strength and control of your pelvic floor muscles, along with bladder training and other behavioral strategies to suppress urgency. In a 237-woman trial comparing the medication tolterodine given alone or with training in behavioral techniques, women receiving the combination achieved better bladder control and were more satisfied with their treatment. However, most were not able to discontinue their medication and sustain the benefits.

■ **Alpha-adrenergic agonists.** Found in some popular cold medicines, these drugs are not designed specifically to treat incontinence. But women with stress incontinence and some men who have undergone prostate removal find these medications help relieve symptoms. Alpha-adrenergic agonists mimic the effects of the neurotransmitter norepinephrine, which, among other things, stimulates the muscles around the bladder neck and urethra to contract and form a tighter seal to keep urine in.

One alpha-adrenergic agonist, pseudoephedrine, is an ingredient in cold and allergy remedies such as some Sudafed formulations. Some people take pseudoephedrine occasionally to minimize stress incontinence. Side effects such as dry mouth and headache may make it unacceptable for everyday use. Also, people with certain medical conditions should not take these types of medications—so ask your doctor before you do so. Although available without a prescription,

---

Going green for tea time

Ordinarily, doctors recommend cutting down on liquids to help control urinary incontinence. But a 2011 study showed that among Japanese women, those who said they drank more green tea had less urinary incontinence than those who drank less tea or none. Women who drank four cups of green tea a day were 66% less likely to report incontinence than those who drank no green tea. Don't get your hopes up for other kinds of tea or coffee, though, as no benefit was seen with anything but green tea. Note that this was a small study of only 298 women. Larger studies are needed to know for sure if green tea actually helps reduce incontinence.

pseudoephedrine-containing products are not stored on open shelves because they can be used in the illegal manufacture of the addictive drug methamphetamine. To purchase, ask the pharmacist or salesperson.

■ **Alpha-adrenergic antagonists.** Alpha-adrenergic antagonists are prescribed to men who develop over-

Table 2 Medications for urinary incontinence

CLASS/GENERIC NAME	BRAND NAME(S)	USE IN INCONTINENCE	SIDE EFFECTS
Alpha-adrenergic agonists			
pseudoephedrine	Sudafed, Trinalin	Stimulates urethral muscle contraction to ease stress incontinence.	Increased heart rate, feelings of unreality, dry mouth, restlessness.
Alpha-adrenergic antagonists			
alfuzosin	Uroxatral	Relax bladder neck muscles in men with obstructions (opens the prostate).	Low blood pressure upon standing up, dizziness, lack of energy, swollen ankles.
doxazosin	Cardura		
tamsulosin	Flomax		
terazosin	Hytrin		
Antibiotics			
several	several	May cure sudden-onset incontinence due to infection.	Side effects vary by drug.
Anticholinergics			
darifenacin	Enablex	Quiet bladder muscle spasms to ease urgency, frequency, and urge incontinence.	Dry mouth, dry eyes, headache, constipation, blurred vision. Slow-release versions cause fewer side effects.
fesoterodine	Toviaz		
flavoxate	Urispas		
oxybutynin	Ditropan XL, Oxytrol patch, generic oxybutynin ER, Gelnique gel		
solifenacin	Vesicare		
tolterodine tartrate	Detrol LA, generic		
trospium	Sanctura and Sanctura XR		
Antidepressants (tricyclic)			
amitriptyline	Elavil	In low doses, may ease overactive bladder and stress incontinence and sometimes nocturia (urinating at night).	Drowsiness, blurry vision, constipation, dry mouth. Many reactions with other medications.
imipramine	Tofranil		
Antidiuretic hormone			
antidiuretic desmopressin	DDAVP, generic	Reduces urine production at night to help nocturia.	Dizziness, headache, weakness, low sodium in blood.
Cholinergic			
bethanechol	Duvoid, Urecholine, generic	Strengthens bladder muscle contraction to treat overflow incontinence.	Shortness of breath, blurry vision, drowsiness.
Injectable neurotoxin			
Botulinum toxin	Botox	Treats overactive bladder and bladder dysfunction caused by nerve damage.	Reduced sensitivity of bladder muscles, urinary retention. Lasts three to 12 months.

flow incontinence when an enlarged prostate interferes with normal urine flow. Also known as alpha blockers, these drugs have the opposite effect of alpha-adrenergic agonists—they relax the smooth muscle of the urethra. They include alfuzosin (Uroxatral), doxazosin (Cardura), tamsulosin (Flomax), and terazosin (Hytrin).

These medications lower blood pressure and may make you prone to a sudden drop in blood pressure when you change position from lying down to sitting or standing (called postural hypotension). To minimize this symptom, your doctor may suggest taking the medication at bedtime. Some doctors are hesitant to prescribe these alpha blockers for men who are already on another blood pressure medication. Other side effects may include dizziness, lack of energy, or swelling of the ankles.

If you are planning cataract surgery, tell your ophthalmologist if you are taking an alpha-adrenergic antagonist. The drugs can affect how the pupils of your eyes act during the procedure, which may necessitate a change in surgical technique.

■ **Anticholinergic medications.** For women, these are the mainstay of treatment for incontinence related to overactive bladder. Anticholinergics block the effects of the neurotransmitter acetylcholine, which causes the detrusor muscle to contract. These are used to quiet the spasms of the bladder muscle that cause frequency, urgency, and urge incontinence.

Anticholinergics such as darifenacin (Enablex), fesoterodine (Toviaz), oxybutynin (Ditropan XL and others), solifenacin (Vesicare), tolterodine tartrate (Detrol LA), and trospium (Sanctura XR) are available in an extended-release form that minimizes side effects. Oxybutynin is also available in topical applications applied to the skin by patch or in gel form. Some people taking the drugs experience side effects such as dry mouth and dry eyes, headache, constipation, and blurred vision. Some older users report memory problems, and the drugs may worsen dementia. Talk to your doctor if you experience side effects or don't get the results you expect. You may need to try more than one medication to discover which works best and causes the fewest side effects. About 80% of people are able to tolerate one of these drugs—a big improvement over older anticholinergics.

You should not use anticholinergics if you have narrow-angle glaucoma, myasthenia gravis, or severe ulcerative colitis. Men should not use the drugs to relieve symptoms in lieu of getting a proper prostate evaluation.

■ **Antidepressants.** An older category of antidepressant drugs known as tricyclic antidepressants can be useful for treating men and women whose primary complaint is that they wake up at night to urinate (a condition called nocturia). Drugs such as amitriptyline (Elavil) and imipramine (Tofranil) combine both anticholinergic and alpha-adrenergic agonist actions. Low doses are sometimes prescribed either alone or in combination with anticholinergics to treat overactive bladder.

Because they can cause drowsiness, these antidepressants can help people sleep through the night without getting up to urinate. Tricyclic antidepressants interact with a number of common medications, so your physician should be aware of all the medications you use (including over-the-counter or alternative remedies) before prescribing them. Antidepressants in the class known as the selective serotonin reuptake inhibitors (SSRIs), such as Prozac, are not effective in treating incontinence.

Duloxetine (Cymbalta) is an antidepressant that inhibits reuptake of both serotonin and norepinephrine. By altering the concentration of these neurotransmitters, the drug seems to increase the contraction of the urethral sphincter. However, this drug is not FDA-approved for the treatment of incontinence, and it is not covered by most health insurance plans when prescribed for urinary incontinence.

■ **Antidiuretic hormone.** This synthetic hormone can be useful for men or women who are primarily troubled by the need to urinate during the night. Vasopressin, an antidiuretic hormone produced by the pituitary gland, signals the kidneys to reduce urine production while you sleep. The synthetic version, called desmopressin (DDAVP), works in the same way. If you have a medical condition that would be worsened by fluid retention (such as high blood pressure or heart failure), your doctor is unlikely to prescribe antidiuretic hormone. Your electrolytes need to be carefully monitored when starting this medication, as it can cause dangerously low levels of sodium in your blood.

■ **Cholinergic medication.** The cholinergic drug bethanechol (Duvoid, Urecholine) strengthens the contractions of the bladder muscle and may be prescribed to men and women who have overflow incontinence because of a weak bladder muscle (not a blockage). Side effects can include shortness of breath, blurry vision, sweating, and dizziness. The medication is usually taken an hour or two before meals to prevent stomach upset. You should not take bethanechol if you have asthma, an overactive thyroid, or Parkinson's disease, or if you have recently had surgery on your urinary system or gastrointestinal tract.

■ **Estrogen.** Estrogen is sometimes prescribed as a vaginal supplement to improve the strength of tissues in the urinary tract of women who show signs of deficiency. It may also help relieve symptoms of urinary frequency and urgency incontinence. However, in the large multicenter trial known as the Women's Health Initiative, oral conjugated equine estrogen (Premarin), both alone and combined with a progestin (as Prempro, the most commonly prescribed formulation), worsened stress incontinence and overactive bladder in postmenopausal women who already had incontinence, and increased the risk that incontinence would develop in women who were continent at the begin-

▶ Choosing a clinician

To get help for incontinence, your primary care physician is a good place to start. But not all physicians have the necessary interest or experience. If your doctor seems unable to help, keep looking. There are several kinds of health professionals and several types of clinics that work with people with these conditions. (For contact information for the organizations mentioned here, see "Resources," page 44.)

Urogynecologists. These are gynecologists who have taken additional training in problems affecting a woman's bladder and pelvis—including urinary and fecal incontinence or prolapse. Check your state's listing on the American Urogynecologic Society Web site. This board-certified subspecialty is also known as Female Pelvic Medicine and Reconstructive Surgery.

Urologists. These medical doctors treat the urinary systems of both men and women as well as the male reproductive organs. The American Urological Association Web site has a physician locator.

Gastroenterologists and colorectal surgeons. These doctors have training in treating conditions of the gastrointestinal tract, including fecal incontinence. If you have diarrhea or digestive symptoms in addition to incontinence, start with a gastroenterologist, particularly if there is no known childbirth injury or other trauma to the sphincter. Several organizations offer physician locators.

Again, keep in mind that not all gastroenterologists have given this problem much attention. In an editorial in the journal *Gastroenterology,* one prominent physician chastised his colleagues for neglecting fecal incontinence.

A colorectal surgeon should be prepared to offer you a range of surgical and nonsurgical options for treatment. The American Society of Colon and Rectal Surgeons has a directory of members.

Anorectal physiology labs. Run by clinicians and equipped to evaluate fecal incontinence, these facilities are often located in hospital departments specializing in motility disorders or functional bowel disorders (most likely gastroenterology, surgery, or urogynecology departments) as well as in some private practices.

Pelvic floor disorders centers. Some hospitals have developed clinics to provide one-stop shopping for the evaluation and treatment of many pelvic floor disorders, including urinary and fecal incontinence. These clinics may combine the expertise of many specialists, including urogynecologists, colorectal surgeons, urologists, gastroenterologists, neurologists, physiatrists (physicians who deal with muscle and skeletal problems and rehabilitation), and physical therapists.

Biofeedback professionals. Health professionals who practice this technique include nurses and physical or occupational therapists. Look for someone with experience in bowel or bladder training. Start by asking the physician treating your incontinence, or contact the Biofeedback Certification Institute of America.

Pelvic floor physical therapists. If you need help learning to strengthen and control your pelvic floor muscles and to use other behavioral strategies to maintain continence, a growing number of physical therapists specialize in this area and have undergone advanced training to earn a Certificate of Achievement of Pelvic Physical Therapy. Ask your physician for a referral, or contact the American Physical Therapy Association.

Nurse specialists. If you are having skin problems related to incontinence or if you have not been able to find acceptable ways to manage your incontinence, a specialist in continence or ostomy nursing can offer practical advice. Contact the Wound, Ostomy, and Continence Nurses Society.

ning of the study. Few studies demonstrate any benefit of vaginal estrogen therapy in treating incontinence. Hormone therapy is generally recommended only for the short-term treatment of menopausal symptoms. However, using vaginal estrogen cream, ring, or suppositories one to three times a week is probably safe over the long term because the estrogen does not enter the bloodstream in significant amounts.

Neurological strategies for overactive bladder

Without your awareness, there is a constant loop of communication between your bladder and one of your lower spinal nerves (the third sacral nerve). About six times per second, the sacral nerve sends an impulse to the bladder to remind it "don't go now." If that signal isn't sufficiently strong or frequent, you can develop problems with urgency and frequency, known as overactive bladder (see page 6). Neurological strategies for overactive bladder attempt to improve the signaling from this sacral nerve.

Sacral neuromodulation

In the late 1990s, the FDA approved a pacemaker-like implanted device for use in men and women with bladder overactivity that has not responded to medication, bladder training, or biofeedback. Since that time, the use of this device has grown more common. If your doctor thinks the device might help you, you can be temporarily fitted with a test system. To do so, the physician places a wire near your sacral nerve and attaches it to an external device that sends electrical impulses through it. This can be done in the physician's office. If your symptoms improve greatly while wearing the device, you are a good candidate for long-term stimulation.

The long-term device is inserted surgically while you are under general or local anesthesia. The surgeon makes a small incision over the sacrum (the spinal bone above your tailbone) and inserts a lead wire there. From the sacrum, the wire runs just under your skin and fat layer until it connects to the small stimulator device (about the size of a stopwatch) implanted just under the skin and fat in an unobtrusive location in your upper buttock or abdomen. You use a handheld control device to adjust the stimulator as necessary. Every three years or so, you will need another minor surgery to replace the battery. The manufacturer warns that it is unsafe to undergo medical treatments involving diathermy (heating parts of the body using electrical currents or ultrasound) while the device is in place; the energy can damage the system and cause serious or life-threatening damage to surrounding tissue. In addition, MRI is not recommended for people with sacral neuromodulation.

On the other hand, this treatment is not without risks. About one-third of patients require repeat surgery because of pain, infection, or movement of the wire. This treatment is expensive, but Medicare and most insurers cover it.

Percutaneous tibial nerve stimulation (PTNS)

A device called the Urgent PC Neuromodulation System takes advantage of the fact that the ankle and the bladder send and receive signals from the same sacral nerve.

For a PTNS treatment, which lasts about half an hour, a hair-thin wire is inserted near the tibial nerve just above your ankle. The wire is connected to an external device that delivers low-frequency electrical pulses. The stimulation travels to the sacral nerve, where it is designed to reset nerve signals to the bladder and thus diminish incontinence related to an overactive bladder. The treatment is used once a week for several weeks and then as needed to control symptoms.

In one U.S. multicenter study, 12 weeks of PTNS treatment cured or improved 80% of patients, compared with 61% of a control group who were prescribed medication (tolterodine).

A person who has both urinary and fecal incontinence may be able to qualify for insurance coverage because the therapy can be billed under urinary incontinence. You should not use this treatment if you are pregnant, have nerve damage, or have a pacemaker or implantable defibrillator.

Botulinum toxin

Best known for its ability to smooth a furrowed brow by paralyzing forehead muscles, this neurotoxin is sometimes used to relieve severe overactive bladder by weakening the detrusor muscle's ability to contract. Your physician passes a cystoscope through the urethra into the bladder, then injects the toxin directly into the detrusor muscle in many locations.

Injection of bulking agents

Injection of a bulking agent can reinforce the tissue around the urethra. This procedure can help some men who have had their prostate removed and some women with the type of stress incontinence known as intrinsic sphincter deficiency, in which the urinary sphincter no longer closes completely and allows urine to leak out, particularly with exertion. After injection, the bulking agent pushes against the urethra to make it narrower, so that it stays closed against increased pressure.

The most common injectables are synthetic polymers and silicone beads, but a variety of different agents are in use. The life span of synthetic bulking agents is unknown, but they have been demonstrated to remain for at least a year.

Injection of bulking agents takes five to 10 minutes and can be performed in the physician's office or as an outpatient procedure in the hospital. Using a cystoscope for viewing, the doctor places a needle into the urethra and injects the bulking agent into the tissue alongside the urethra. A few injections may be given during one session. Although the procedure is minimally invasive and can be considered nonsurgical, you will be given either local anesthesia, a light general anesthesia, or sedation. Only small amounts of bulking agents are injected at one time, so more than one treatment may be needed to achieve satisfactory results. Physicians must be cautious about injecting too much, as this can cause inability to urinate.

For the first day or two after an injection, you may feel irritation when you urinate. You might even need to use a catheter to drain the bladder intermittently until swelling goes down in the area of the injection. After a few days, you should be able to return to normal activities.

Bulking agents work best in women with intrinsic sphincter deficiency; it is not likely to help if you have overactive bladder, an abnormally small bladder capacity, or a bladder neck that is hypermobile (not well supported). In general, bulking agents are most useful for older women who, are not physically active and who may not be good candidates for other treatments. They don't work as well as other methods, particularly in people who are physically active. About 80% of women show some level of improvement; 40% become dry and remain dry with only one or two treatments.

Some men have this procedure after prostate removal; the bulking agent is injected into the area the prostate had occupied in order to provide support for the urethral muscles, so urine isn't as easily lost. Although 70% of men experience some improvement in their symptoms, only 8% become dry with one or two treatments and require no further injections.

You should not be injected with bulking agents if you have a urinary tract infection or have had many in the past, or if the physician sees through the cystoscope that the lining of your urethra is fragile and might erode in the area of the injection.

Surgery

The trend in surgery for incontinence is toward less invasive surgical procedures that can usually be performed on an outpatient basis and sometimes in the physician's office. Because some surgical procedures for stress incontinence are now relatively quick and require less recovery time, your doctor may recommend surgery earlier if your incontinence is caused by a repairable structural problem or if it seems unlikely that nonsurgical approaches will be satisfactory. When choosing to have minimally invasive surgery, it is especially important that your surgeon be highly trained and experienced in the specific procedure you choose.

The most common condition treated surgically is stress incontinence; this is done by inserting a sling of material to support the urethra. Overactive bladder may also be treated with the surgical implantation of a neuromodulation device (see "Sacral neuromodulation," page 23). If incontinence is caused by a prolapsed uterus in a woman or an enlarged prostate in a man, surgery to correct those conditions (not described in this report) may relieve the incontinence along with other symptoms.

Whether and when to have surgery is a personal decision that has no right or wrong answer. You may consider surgery if nonsurgical treatments are not providing the control you need or if an anatomical problem makes it unlikely that nonsurgical techniques will help. Even if surgery is ultimately your choice, the effort you spend in bladder training and strengthening your pelvic muscles is not wasted; these techniques increase the chance of a successful outcome following surgery for incontinence and can reduce postoperative incontinence after prostate surgery. After their operations, some people say they regret the time they spent coping with incontinence and wish they had taken the step sooner. Others hope to put off the decision as long as possible, because new and less invasive procedures are becoming available every year.

Surgery for stress incontinence

For women, surgeries for stress incontinence are designed to provide extra support for the urethra so it can remain closed under physical stress, such as during coughing or sneezing. This can be done by several methods. For years, the best method was the Burch procedure, a form of bladder neck suspension in which the surgeon places stitches on either side of the urethra and bladder neck and attaches the stitches to a ligament at the top of the pubic bone. Now, the most common procedure involves a simple-to-install sling of synthetic mesh that supports the urethra, hammock-style.

Before you and your doctor decide on surgery, you may need to have detailed diagnostic testing (see "Evaluating urinary incontinence," page 8) to help determine which type of surgery would work best. The availability of minimally invasive procedures has led physicians to consider such treatments for stress incontinence in women who are younger and have less severe incontinence as well as older women who may benefit from a minimally invasive procedure. However, women who hope to have future pregnancies are often advised to postpone surgery if possible until childbearing is complete, because delivering a baby through the vaginal canal may undo the effects of the surgery. If you do choose surgery, choose your surgeon and procedure carefully, because additional attempts may be less successful.

Before your surgery, gain the best control possible over your bladder by strengthening your pelvic floor, using bladder training, and avoiding bladder irritants such as caffeine. This will minimize urinary urgency and frequency that sometimes develop following surgery.

Three distressing but uncommon problems may occur after any type of surgery for stress incontinence, although the risks vary with the different procedures:

- You might develop symptoms of overactive bladder, even if you were never troubled by them before (7% to 15% of patients experience this).
- Although it's not common, you might undo the benefits of the surgery by lifting or other strenuous activity, even after the healing period is over.
- You might go from incontinence to having difficulty urinating temporarily, in rare cases requiring a catheter to empty your bladder.
- The mesh sling may erode or perforate vaginal or other tissues.

▪ **Sling and tape procedures.** These procedures have become increasingly common because they are less invasive and equally effective compared with older surgical methods, such as the Burch procedure discussed below. For these procedures, a surgeon installs a supportive sling under and around the urethra to support it. The sling is made of either your own tissue or an artificial tape similar to nylon or polypropylene, common materials used for sutures. In women, the sling can support the urethra in the proper position, which helps the urethra hold in urine during a cough or sneeze. In 2011, the FDA issued a safety recommendation warning doctors and their female patients that installing a mesh sling to treat pelvic organ prolapse has resulted in complications such as erosion of the vaginal wall, pain, and bleeding. The FDA is reviewing the rate of complications for the sling for urinary incontinence. If you are considering one of these procedures, the key to a successful, complication-free outcome is choosing an experienced surgeon who performs the procedure frequently.

In men, the sling puts pressure on the urethra just below the bladder.

After less invasive surgery such as this, recovery is rapid. If you are over age 70 or have other medical problems, you may be hospitalized overnight. Otherwise, you will probably be discharged after you have recovered from any anesthesia and have been able to urinate. You may need pain relief medication for a few days. Initially your urine stream may be slower. When you sit to urinate, relax and wait for the reflex that starts urine flowing. Straining can make it more difficult to urinate and can loosen the sling.

■ **For women.** Two types of minimally invasive sling surgery are available. In one, known as a transvaginal tape (TVT) procedure, the surgeon places a hammock of narrow mesh underneath the urethra and extending up to two anchors in the abdominal wall above the pubic bone, forming a *U*-shape to support the urethra (see Figure 6). The mesh stays in place without sutures, as your body creates scar tissue around and through the mesh. This surgery (available in several systems with brand names such as Gynecare TVT and SPARC) is faster and easier than older, more invasive sling procedures and, in many cases, can be performed under local anesthesia. Some surgeons combine the placement of TVT with other pelvic reconstructive surgery, such as vaginal hysterectomy or repair of cystocele or rectocele (bladder or rectal tissues bulging into the vagina). Most women can return to work within three to seven days after a TVT sling procedure as long as no heavy lifting is required at work.

In a second minimally invasive sling procedure, transobturator tape (TOT, with brand names such as Monarc and Uratape) is inserted through a small vaginal incision, and the ends are brought out through tiny incisions between the labia and the creases of the thighs. The sling supports the urethra gently, forming a curve shaped more like a smile than the letter U. No sutures or anchors are used. Surgery takes about half an hour, and most women can return to work within a few days if they do not have to lift heavy objects. Performed without an abdominal incision, this procedure reduces the risk of bowel or bladder injury during surgery, and it can be used in women who have scar tissue from previous surgeries.

The field continues to evolve as ever less invasive procedures are developed. A newer, single-incision sling procedure, called the mini sling, involves inserting a supportive mesh hammock under the urethra using a slim needle. The procedure requires a small vaginal incision but no abdominal or groin incisions, and it can be performed in an outpatient surgery center or a physician's office under local anesthesia. Since the mini sling was introduced in 2007, preliminary research results have shown it is as effective as the regular slings. No long-term data on its effectiveness are yet available.

In all sling and tape procedures, it is important that patients follow postoperative instructions to avoid excessive activity, such as lifting or exercise, after the sling is in place. After the surgery, there is a possibility that the sling will push too hard against the urethra, blocking the flow of urine. If this occurs, a second, minor surgery may be necessary to loosen up the sling. Some people develop symptoms of urinary urgency (even if this was never a problem previously) that can usually be controlled with medication, bladder training, or Kegel exercises.

■ **For men.** Minimally invasive sling surgery (also called bulbourethral sling surgery, or by brand names such as AdVance and InVance) is relatively simple and usually does not require an overnight hospital stay. During the half-hour procedure, which is performed under spinal or general anesthesia, the surgeon makes

Figure 6 Sling surgery (for women)

For some women with stress incontinence (leaking when coughing or jumping), the surgical insertion of a urethral sling or tape can help support the urethra. In the version shown here, known as a transvaginal tape (TVT) procedure, the surgeon makes a small incision under the urethra through the vagina and two small incisions in the lower abdomen, to insert a strip of synthetic mesh under the urethra to support it. Gradually, your body's own tissues grow through the mesh to hold it in place.

an incision between the scrotum and rectum and attaches the sling to anchors or screws inserted into each side of the pelvic bone.

Complications following male sling procedures can include infection, discomfort, and a shift from incontinence to the opposite problem—difficulty urinating and urinary retention. Men may need to use a catheter to empty their bladders for a short time after this surgery. The sling is usually for men who have mild to moderate stress incontinence due to prostate removal or treatment, other surgery, or trauma. Scarring from previous surgeries or injuries (such as a pelvic fracture) may decrease the likelihood of success.

■ **Bladder neck suspension.** This procedure, known as the Burch colposuspension, has been largely replaced by the sling and tape procedures discussed above. Bladder neck suspension is a surgical procedure for women with stress incontinence that elevates or increases support for the bladder neck area to protect against leakage when a woman coughs or exerts herself physically. This operation often involves cutting an incision of three to five inches in the lower abdomen and lifting the tissue next to the bladder neck up, using strong stitches (sutures) to anchor the tissue to a ligament (called Cooper's ligament) near the pubic bone. The Burch procedure is performed under general anesthesia and usually requires a two-day hospital stay and six weeks of recovery before a woman can return to full activity. Sometimes the procedure can be performed laparoscopically, with a quicker recovery.

Surgery for overflow incontinence

If you have overflow incontinence because something is blocking your urethra (such as an enlarged prostate in a man) or bladder (such as a prolapsed uterus in a woman), surgery can be performed to remove the obstruction. The procedures and results will depend on the exact cause and location of the blockage.

For example, a man with an enlarged prostate may undergo transurethral resection of the prostate, or TURP, an incision-free surgical procedure that reduces prostate tissues with an electrical loop. It relieves urinary obstruction in at least 75% of cases, and the improvement is usually long-lasting. However, urinary problems can recur if the prostate tissue grows back. While TURP may aid overflow incontinence, other types of incontinence may occur as a side effect of the procedure.

Women with incontinence resulting from a prolapsed bladder, uterus, or rectum may undergo procedures to reposition the out-of-place organs and shore up their support.

Artificial urinary sphincter

An artificial sphincter is a fluid-filled cuff surgically placed around the urethra to prevent urine from leaking out (see Figure 7). A small pump is inserted into a woman's labium or a man's scrotum. To urinate, you squeeze the pump and the fluid drains from the cuff into a storage balloon implanted in the abdominal cavity. This releases pressure on the urethra and allows urine to flow out. Over the next few minutes, the fluid automatically returns to the cuff.

The operation to implant the cuff, balloon, and pump takes about two hours and three small incisions. It is usually performed under general anesthe-

Figure 7 Artificial urinary sphincter (for men)

For men who have had prostate surgery, initial incontinence usually improves over several months. But for those with intractable incontinence caused by sphincter weakness, the artificial sphincter is a possible solution. After it is surgically inserted, the fluid-filled cuff compresses the urethra to stop the flow of urine. To allow urination, a man squeezes a small pump to open the cuff and allow urine to pass. The cuff automatically refills.

▶ **Selecting your procedure and surgeon**

If you are planning surgery for urinary incontinence, you may have several choices of procedures. Among the factors in your decision will be the risks and benefits of each option and the specific problems your evaluation has revealed. In addition, you and your physician may favor one approach over another for individual reasons. Among things to consider: Is a rapid recovery and return to work a priority? Do you need another pelvic surgery—such as a hysterectomy, tubal ligation, or treatment for prolapse—that can be done at the same time? Are you more comfortable using your own tissue or a synthetic?

In the rapidly changing field of incontinence surgery, not all surgeons may be prepared to offer the least invasive option suitable to your medical situation. Look for a urologist or urogynecologist who has substantial experience in urinary procedures, is adept at cystoscopy (since the surgeon must use a lighted medical scope to inspect the inside of the bladder at the end of most procedures), and is up to date with the latest approaches.

---

sia. During a healing period of four to six weeks, the pump will not be activated. Once the pump is activated, your urinary control will improve. The major complications with an artificial sphincter include the possibility of infection, erosion of the tissue around the implants, or malfunctioning or shifting of the device. Such complications may require surgery to repair or remove the device.

Artificial sphincters are used far less frequently in women than in men. However, if you are a woman with severe stress incontinence due to intrinsic sphincter deficiency, or if you are still having major leakage problems after other surgeries, the artificial sphincter is an option.

Suprapubic tube insertion

For severe and intractable incontinence, a surgeon can insert a suprapubic (above the pubic bone) tube from outside your abdomen directly into your bladder. Urine is diverted through the tube and collected in a bag outside the body. Although this solution is a last resort, it is easier than other management techniques for people in some situations. Although for the average person this would mean a decrease in quality of life, for those with truly severe incontinence, it can be a big improvement. ▼

Managing urinary incontinence

Many people must cope with urinary incontinence—at least for a while before treatment, and sometimes afterward as well, if treatment does not completely correct the symptoms. If you are experiencing urinary incontinence, even temporarily, it's important to realize that you have other options beyond the expensive pads and "adult diapers" available on drugstore shelves. There are options designed specifically for men or women as well as pad-and-pants systems tailored to specific types of incontinence.

If you must deal with incontinence, seek advice from health professionals or support organizations such as the National Association for Continence (see "Resources," page 44). You will find less expensive, more effective products and learn strategies to maximize your ability to work, travel, and participate in your favorite activities. You can also learn about ways to help prevent your problem from worsening (see "Preventing urinary or fecal incontinence," page 30).

Containment options

A tremendous variety of pads and other absorbent products are available to suit your sex and the type or severity of your incontinence. In general, products designated for "light" protection will absorb up to one cup; "moderate," up to two cups; and "heavy," up to three cups.

When choosing a pad, look for products specifically for incontinence that incorporate superabsorbent layers; these pull fluid away from the skin into the core of the pad, where it forms a gel that can't leak out. Look for such brand names as Tena Serenity, Poise, and Depend. Check with your insurer about coverage for products to manage incontinence. If your insurance does not cover these products, some people find they can use less-expensive children's diapers.

■ **For women.** Products include a range of disposable and reusable pads and underwear. Among these are traditional underwear designs with a special crotch that wicks urine away from the surface and stores it. If you are limited in movement and dexterity, ask about products that are designed for easy use by people with disabilities. Women with mild incontinence may use less expensive and readily available menstrual pads, reserving specific (more expensive) incontinence products for when extra protection and dryness are needed. Before investing in a large quantity of incontinence pads, try smaller packages of several brands to see which works best for you; many women strongly prefer one brand over another.

■ **For men.** There are several absorbent products designed with the male anatomy in mind. Drip shields (with light protection) or guards (that absorb more) with waterproof backings slip over the head of the penis and can be kept in place with any relatively tight-fitting briefs. Some cover the scrotum as well and fit better if the penis is small or retracted. Brand names include Attends and Conveen. These products absorb 3 to 4 ounces of urine. When men with light incontinence compared four types of products, drip guards were the favored design for day and night use. For heavier incontinence, you can wear absorbent inserts, shaped to fit men (such as Depend and Dignity), inside your own underwear or special mesh briefs.

Collection devices

When there is constant leakage, devices that collect rather than absorb the urine can help to protect the

Is your home making things worse?

Falling on the way to the bathroom can cause fracture or other injury, particularly for someone with overactive bladder or someone who gets up at night to urinate.

One solution is a bedside commode. Other steps that can prevent falls include installing grab bars and nonslip surfaces in the bathroom, wearing flat-soled slippers or shoes that grip well, and clearing throw rugs and obstacles from the path between your bed and the bathroom.

skin. The National Association for Continence advises you to seek professional guidance in selecting the type and size that would work best for you. Otherwise, you may conclude that a device is unsatisfactory when the problem may, in fact, lie in its fit or style.

■ **For men.** Men can choose from a variety of external devices. A condom catheter, also known as a "Texas catheter," is a soft sheath made of silicone or latex that fits over the penis like a regular condom, except that it attaches to a drain tube leading to a urine collection

Preventing urinary or fecal incontinence

Not all incontinence is avoidable. But there are some lifestyle choices you can make that reduce the risk of developing either urinary or fecal incontinence.

Maintain a healthy weight. Particularly for women, obesity is linked with incontinence. In people with obesity, the pelvic floor muscles must support excess abdominal fat as well as the pelvic organs, which can lead to stress incontinence. In addition, obesity may place pressure on the bladder and interfere with its blood and nerve supply. Fat tissue itself may contribute to overactive bladder by altering the balance of chemical messengers between nerve cells. Weight loss can sometimes improve incontinence without other treatment.

A connection between obesity and urinary incontinence is less well-documented in men. However, in some surveys, obese men report more urinary tract symptoms, including urgency and nocturia, and they are more likely to require surgery for an enlarged prostate (a procedure that sometimes leads to incontinence).

For men as well as women, many surgeries to counter incontinence are less successful in those who are obese.

Don't smoke. Smoking nearly doubles the likelihood that a woman will develop stress incontinence, perhaps because it can lead to frequent and violent coughing. Compared with other incontinent women, female smokers develop incontinence at a younger age, despite having relatively stronger sphincter muscles. Nicotine has also been linked to urge incontinence. In studies involving men, current or former smoking is associated with several bothersome urinary symptoms, including urge incontinence, but the increase in risk (about 39%) is not as striking as that for stress incontinence in women.

Stay active. High-impact exercises (such as jumping jacks) or specific maneuvers (such as a golf swing) can elicit leakage if you have stress incontinence. But don't let fear of leaks keep you from being physically active. In the Nurses' Health Study, middle-aged women who were most physically active were least likely to develop incontinence.

Minimize bladder irritants. Several foods have been linked to urge incontinence. Caffeine and alcohol are diuretics that result in rapid filling of the bladder and a powerful urge to urinate, even when the bladder is not full. Carbonated drinks, the artificial sweetener aspartame (NutraSweet), spicy foods, and citrus fruits and juices cause urgency in some people.

Don't ignore the call. When you get your body's signal that the rectum is full, it's normal to wait until you can conveniently reach a bathroom. But when you routinely put off having a bowel movement as long as possible, it can lead to constipation and ultimately to urinary or fecal incontinence.

Don't strain with bowel movements. Years of forcing can weaken a man's or a woman's pelvic floor muscles. Even when you have regular bowel movements, if your stools are frequently hard or take considerable effort to pass, you have constipation and could benefit from medical advice. In a study involving people ages 65 and older, treating constipation improved a variety of urinary symptoms, including frequency, urgency, and burning. Increasing the fiber in your diet and drinking adequate fluids can help prevent constipation.

Consider incontinence when making medical decisions. When you are considering any type of pelvic or abdominal surgery, such as a hysterectomy, prostate removal, or treatment for hemorrhoids (painful swellings in the anus) or anal fistula (a painful crack or slit in the anus), ask about the risk for subsequent incontinence for the proposed procedure and its alternatives. For example, prostate removal may result in urinary stress incontinence (an estimated 14% of men still have frequent urine leakage five years after the procedure), but alternative treatment with radiation seed therapy may cause urge incontinence, and external beam radiation can lead to bowel problems, including fecal incontinence. When a medication is prescribed, inquire about incontinence as a possible side effect and whether alternatives are available if symptoms occur.

If you are pregnant, ask your obstetrician about how often episiotomies are used in vaginal deliveries in that practice, and under what circumstances (see "The childbirth connection," page 5). If episiotomy is used frequently or routinely, discuss your concerns about sphincter damage and seek another practitioner if needed.

Get help early. Early symptoms are a warning sign. Don't wait for symptoms to worsen. Report symptoms to your doctor. Ask to see a pelvic floor physical therapist who can work with you to strengthen or stabilize your pelvic floor muscles to regain bladder and bowel control and improve your quality of life.

bag, usually worn on the leg. Some condom catheters are self-adhesive; others must be strapped on, held in place with a jockstrap, or taped on with adhesive strips. Some are reusable, and others, disposable.

The major concern in using a condom catheter is protecting your skin. Usually, you should clean and dry your penis and apply a moisture-protective cream before attaching a new condom catheter. Some men develop a sensitivity to latex and should choose a silicone catheter.

■ **For women.** A few urine collection pouches (such as Hollister) are designed to be held around the opening to the urethra with adhesive or suction. The end of the pouch is connected to a larger drainage bag so you can move around freely.

Clamps for men

For men, an alternative to pads or collection devices is a clamp placed around the base of the penis and tightened just enough to prevent urine from leaking. The device is designed as an inflatable ring or a foam-lined metal or plastic frame. Every couple of hours, you loosen the clamp to urinate and keep pressure from building up. Whether a clamp works will depend on whether you can adjust it to prevent leakage and still remain comfortable. If you have damaged skin on the penis, are physically unable to loosen the clamp yourself, or have nerve damage that might make it difficult for you to judge the clamp's tightness, you could damage the tissues of the penis and are better off choosing a different method. Penile clamps are available without a prescription (brand names include Bard Cunningham), but may be covered by Medicare or your private insurer if ordered through your physician.

Clean intermittent catheterization

If you are a man or woman with overflow incontinence because your bladder muscles are weak or your bladder does not completely empty for other reasons, such as complications of surgery for incontinence, you may be able to manage the situation with intermittent self-catheterization. For this approach, you urinate normally every few hours, trying to empty your bladder as completely as possible. Next you insert a small tube (the catheter) through the urethra into the bladder to drain any remaining urine into the toilet.

Although it may sound difficult, this technique is a major advance for people who need temporary or permanent help urinating. The procedure is not usually painful, and you do not need to keep the catheter sterile or use gloves. Urinary tract infections can be a problem, but this technique poses a smaller risk than a permanent catheter would.

Pessaries for women

For centuries, women have used a device called a pessary, placed inside the vagina in a manner similar to a contraceptive diaphragm. A pessary is designed to hold a prolapsed bladder or uterus in place; in the process, it can help prevent urine leakage by supporting the urethra. Although it sounds old-fashioned and doesn't actually repair the problem, a pessary can

Dribble relief

Many men, young and old, are troubled by the dribbling of urine after the main stream has stopped and the bladder feels empty. Even if they wait a moment and shake the penis before zipping up, there can be embarrassing wet or stained trousers. At highest risk: men with enlarged prostates.

The medical term for this is post-micturition dribbling. It occurs when the muscles surrounding the urethra don't squeeze hard enough for it to empty completely, leaving a small pool of urine at a dip in the urethra behind the base of the penis. Within a few minutes, the urine dribbles out.

Try these approaches to avoid wet and stained trousers:

- Practice pelvic floor exercises to increase muscle strength.
- "Milk out" the last few drops of urine. Using the fingertips of one hand, start about an inch behind your scrotum, and gently press upward. Keep applying this pressure as you move your fingers toward the base of the penis under the scrotum. Repeat. This maneuver should move the pooled urine into the penis, where you can shake out the last few drops. With practice, you should be able to do this quickly and unobtrusively.

In women, dribbling can occur when a little urine gets trapped in the vagina, dripping out when you stand up from the toilet. Wipe inside the vagina before standing to see if this eliminates the dripping.

mimic the benefit of a surgical bladder neck suspension and is a very practical solution for some women with prolapse that results in stress incontinence.

Pessaries are usually ring- or dish-shaped and are available only through a physician or other health care provider. The pessary must be fitted by your health care provider to support the bladder neck properly when it is inserted. Your clinician may suggest you use a pessary while you wait for surgery. This device might also be an option if surgery is considered medically unsafe or unlikely to relieve your symptoms, if you develop stress incontinence while pregnant, or if you prefer a nonsurgical option. But it's usually not helpful if you have overactive bladder. If you have a vaginal infection, that will have to be treated before you use a pessary.

Whether you find a pessary beneficial will depend largely on your anatomy. If your pessary fits properly (and it typically takes two or more tries to select the ideal size and style), it should not fall out during normal activities and should not interfere with regular urination or having a bowel movement. Some pessaries can be left in place during intercourse, although you may be more comfortable removing it. A health professional can work with you until you are comfortable inserting the device and removing it for cleaning. Some pessaries must be removed every few days; others can be left in place for several months and are removed for cleaning at regular medical visits.

Skin care

When incontinence is ongoing, it can be a challenge to keep the skin clean and healthy. Skin irritation can be an annoyance in some people, but it may become a serious medical problem in others who develop pressure sores. Urine is particularly irritating because it is acidic; this increases the possibility that you will develop erosion of the skin. You can avoid skin irritation with measures to properly cleanse, repair, and protect the skin.

In general, after each episode of incontinence, cleanse the area with tepid water or a gentle, nonalkaline soap or cleanser. Then protect the skin with a lotion or cream used to protect baby skin, such as Desitin, or specifically developed for incontinence. Avoid products with alcohol or propylene glycol, which can irritate the skin or cause an allergic reaction.

For more information, go to the Web site of the National Association for Continence at www.nafc.org.

Odor control

An unpleasant urine smell can interfere with your work and social activities. But simple changes in your normal routine can prevent or minimize odors.

If you don't drink much fluid, a strong odor may mean your urine is too concentrated. If so, drinking more water may help. But don't go overboard, or you might increase leakage. Acidic urine tends to have less odor, so you can take extra ascorbic acid (vitamin C) or cranberry juice to lower your urine's pH. Certain foods, such as asparagus, may add odor to the urine. A strong odor to the urine may also be a sign of urinary tract infection.

Urine collection devices can be cleaned with plain white vinegar and water, and you can add vinegar or baking soda to your wash water to remove a urine smell from clothing. Vinegar is much better at eliminating odors than products that attempt to cover odors with heavy fragrances.

Emotional concerns

Whether your incontinence is mild or severe, you may be coping with a range of unpleasant emotions stemming from the condition—fear, embarrassment, anxiety, shame, loneliness, and depression.

Although you may feel quite isolated, help is available from many sources. Just getting medical treatment for incontinence has been shown to improve psychological well-being, whether or not the symptoms dramatically improve.

Consider seeking help from a therapist—particularly one familiar with incontinence. A therapist can help you cope with your emotions and with the rigors and uncertainties of treatment. And don't be afraid to tell friends and family. You'd be surprised how many other people, male and female, have experienced some form of incontinence. A support group can link you to others who are going through the same experience and can offer practical advice and emotional support.

Fecal incontinence

Fecal incontinence is the unintended passage of stool. Both men and women may experience such leakage, but it is more common in women, particularly those who have given birth. For both men and women, the incidence of fecal incontinence increases with age, as connective tissues and muscles of the pelvic floor weaken.

Until recently, experts could only guess at how often this condition affected men and women. But for the first time, national statistics have been collected, at least for women, by the National Center for Health Statistics. A survey of 1,961 women, published in 2008, found that at least 9% of women experience the unintended leakage of stool at least once a month.

If you have fecal incontinence, you may not be able to hold in your stool long enough to reach the bathroom. Or you might experience unexpected leakage of stool when you haven't felt any urge (see Figure 8). The symptoms of fecal incontinence can range from mild occasional leakage of liquid stool to a daily debilitating condition with consequences for self-confidence, self-image, and the ability to maintain friendships or careers. Most people with fecal incontinence don't tell their friends, families, or even their doctors. Instead, they limit their activities to avoid accidents and embarrassment. This can result in isolation and depression.

Because people are reluctant to seek help, fecal incontinence is sometimes perceived as rare. This perception is wrong. Fecal incontinence occurs in adults of all ages, and for older or disabled people, it is a leading reason for nursing home placement. One survey found that nearly half of nursing home residents had fecal incontinence.

Fecal incontinence often goes hand in hand with urinary incontinence. Even though they may not disclose it readily, many people with urinary incontinence have fecal incontinence as well.

Most people with fecal incontinence can be helped. If you or someone you know is experiencing fecal incontinence, seek medical advice. There are new options for evaluating, treating, and managing this distressing condition, and even if your previous attempts to get help have been unsatisfactory, you may be able to get help now. While available treatments may not completely cure fecal incontinence, they can lead to gradual improvements that increase quality of life and allow a patient to participate more fully in daily activities.

Anatomy of fecal continence

You rely on your digestive system to process the food you eat. The system absorbs vital nutrients into the bloodstream, and then removes the remaining waste

Figure 8 Causes of fecal incontinence

A. Pelvic floor damage
B. Nerve damage (pudendal nerve)
C. Prolapsed rectum
D. Sphincter damage

Surgery, constipation, radiation treatments, childbirth in women, and other causes contribute to fecal incontinence. For example, surgery may cause damage to pelvic floor muscles (A) or pudendal nerves (B). Chronic diarrhea or constipation can damage the rectum (C). Childbirth or surgery can damage the anal sphincters (D).

products and indigestible food components from your body. By the time food has traveled through your digestive tract to your large intestine, or colon, it is made up of waste material, which continues to lose water and solidify as it slowly moves along. The final product is known as stool, or feces.

At the end of your digestive tract are two areas crucial to fecal continence: the rectum and the anal canal. Muscles in the colon propel feces into the rectum, which has walls that stretch to hold the stool. The last inch of the rectum is called the anal canal. Two kinds of muscle surround it. The internal anal sphincter, which is not under your conscious control, stays contracted most of the time to prevent leakage. The external anal sphincter surrounds the internal anal sphincter.

How does your body know when to release stool? You have stretch-detecting nerve endings in the rectum. When your nerves detect that the rectum is full, the internal sphincter opens briefly and lets a tiny bit of the rectum's contents come in contact with the external sphincter, which is rich with nerve endings. In a rapid "sampling reflex," these nerves inform the brain about whether the rectal contents are intestinal gas or liquid or solid stool. This allows you to act accordingly. You might allow gas to escape, or look for a bathroom right away if you have diarrhea. Otherwise, you might decide whether it is convenient to have a bowel movement, or whether you want to wait for a better time or place.

To delay, you tighten the external anal sphincter (usually without thinking about it) to hold feces inside. As you are attempting to hold in stool, you also contract the puborectalis muscle, a pelvic floor muscle that loops around the rectum. When this muscle is contracted, it pulls the rectum so that it lies at a 90-degree angle to the anal canal rather than more directly above it. This counters the pull of gravity. Contracting these muscles often curbs the urge to defecate. The urge returns when more feces enter the rectum.

Once you are in the bathroom, you relax the puborectalis muscle and both the internal and external sphincters. Then, to propel the stool downward, you increase pressure in the abdominal cavity through the Valsalva or "bearing down" maneuver—closing off the airway, tightening the abdominal muscles, and pushing the diaphragm down.

What can go wrong?

Fecal incontinence is a symptom, not a disease. It can result if something goes wrong with any of the coordinated mechanisms that help maintain continence. The problem is not always caused by a malfunction in the gastrointestinal tract. In some situations, functional incontinence occurs when an unrelated condition, such as arthritis, makes it physically difficult to reach the toilet. In other situations, incontinence involves the malfunction of the bowel or rectum. This kind of incontinence usually stems from one of several common causes.

■ **Bowel problems.** Even if your rectum and anal canal are functioning properly, the system can be overwhelmed by conditions that speed the passage of waste products through the colon, resulting in diarrhea. For example, you may have incontinence temporarily during a bout of food poisoning or in reaction to a medication.

Conditions that cause chronic diarrhea, such as irritable bowel syndrome and inflammatory bowel disease, can lead to occasional or ongoing problems with fecal incontinence. Diabetes may cause nighttime diarrhea that is difficult to control. Sometimes people with minor sphincter damage (see below) are able to maintain continence for a long time. But years after the damage, a bowel problem may develop that stresses the sphincters and ends their control.

■ **Reduced rectal capacity.** Surgery, pelvic radiation (to treat cancer of the prostate or uterus), or inflammatory bowel disease can stiffen or scar the rectum. Then the rectum loses elasticity and cannot store a normal amount of stool. You will have less time between the sensation of stool being present and an urgent need to find a toilet. Diarrhea is particularly difficult to hold.

■ **Constipation.** When hard fecal matter becomes stuck in the rectum, constipation or impaction may occur, causing liquid stool to eventually leak out around the hardened stool. This type of fecal incontinence is called overflow incontinence. It can be confused with diarrhea, but antidiarrheal medications only make the situation worse.

■ **Sphincter damage.** If the internal anal sphincter is damaged, bits of stool can leak out without you being aware of it or able to control it. This may occur at times of physical exertion or after you have had a bowel movement. If, on the other hand, the external anal sphincter muscles are damaged, you may be unable to squeeze hard enough or long enough to make it to the toilet. While you are rushing to the bathroom, incontinence may occur. In women, the most common cause of sphincter injury is vaginal childbirth. The risk increases if a woman has a large baby; is older at the time of delivery; or has a long second stage of labor (pushing), a forceps delivery, a tear that extends to the anus, or an episiotomy (an incision to extend the vaginal opening in an attempt to avoid a tear). Sometimes fecal incontinence is apparent immediately after childbirth. Other times, when less severe sphincter damage occurs, symptoms of incontinence do not appear until decades later. The anal sphincters can also be damaged during rectal surgery (to treat prolapse, hemorrhoids, malformations, or rectal cancer), traumatic injury, or forceful anal intercourse.

■ **Pelvic floor muscle weakness and thinning.** Fecal incontinence can result if your pelvic floor muscles become weak, or if they contract and relax at inappropriate times. Pelvic floor weakness might result from vaginal deliveries or years of straining to defecate.

■ **Rectal prolapse.** When the muscles supporting the rectum are weak, the rectal lining may descend into the anal canal or even protrude from the body. (Hemorrhoids are not rectal prolapse.) If you have a rectal prolapse, you may feel an urgent need to go even when little stool is present. Your external sphincter must work harder to keep you continent. Most people with rectal prolapse have some degree of fecal incontinence. Untreated rectal prolapse can cause long-term stretching and damage of the sphincter, so it is important to seek treatment if you notice any sign of rectal tissue emerging from the anus.

■ **Nerve damage.** If nerves controlling the sphincters malfunction, proper muscle action is impaired, and incontinence may develop. If sensory nerves are damaged, it becomes difficult to perceive that there is stool in the rectum. The pudendal nerve is the major nerve supplying the external sphincter. Damage to this nerve, resulting in incontinence, can occur when the pelvic floor muscles are stretched or traumatized by childbirth or repeated straining to defecate, or if a person develops a neurological condition (such as multiple sclerosis, stroke, diabetic neuropathy, or spinal cord injury).

■ **Rectocele.** In women, the rectum may bulge into the vagina because of weakening of the vaginal wall. This can be caused by vaginal childbirth. Some women find it helps to place one or more fingers inside the vagina when having a bowel movement, to help support the bulging tissue. Rectocele is not considered to be a direct cause of fecal incontinence, but it is sometimes associated with intussusception, the first stage of rectal prolapse (see left) which can cause either incontinence or constipation.

Evaluating fecal incontinence

A surprising number of people with fecal incontinence don't seek medical attention. Half of those with severe incontinence and 95% of people with occasional accidents try to cope on their own and therefore miss getting the help that is available. Your primary care physician is likely to be a good place to start, but don't be surprised if you are referred to a specialist for evaluation (see "Choosing a clinician," page 22). Ideally, your physicians will work together to arrive at the best approach to the problem.

Talking to your doctor about fecal incontinence can be embarrassing. Keep in mind that, to your physician, fecal incontinence is not a personal problem, but a medical symptom like any other—one that needs to be investigated thoroughly because there are so many possible causes. To that end, you can help by being prepared to answer detailed questions:

• When did the incontinence start?

• How often do you have an accident? What happens? Do you lose a large or small amount of stool? Do you have any warning? Does anything seem to bring it on (such as physical activity, stress, time in menstrual cycle, particular foods)?

• Is it getting worse over time? Does anything seem to make it better or worse?

• When your rectum is full, can you distinguish whether it is solid, liquid, or gas? Do you sometimes think you are passing gas, only to be surprised that stool has come out?

- When you feel the need to have a bowel movement, how long can you wait?
- After you defecate, do you feel like there is stool left inside?
- What are your regular bowel habits? Do you often have diarrhea or constipation? Do you often have cramps or see blood in your stool?
- Are you using pads or other means to manage the incontinence? How is it working?
- Do you use any products to prevent constipation?
- Do you also experience urinary incontinence?

Because a wide variety of medical conditions and injuries can affect continence (and the symptoms may not appear until much later), the doctor will need a detailed medical history. If you have delivered one or more babies, it may be helpful to tell the doctor about the length of your labors, how much the babies weighed, whether deliveries involved the use of forceps or episiotomies, whether you had any tears that needed repair, and how your bowels functioned after the deliveries.

Let the physician know about other medical conditions you have and any medications (over-the-counter or prescription) you take. Also relevant are any injuries or treatments in your pelvic region. For example, have you had prostate or hemorrhoid surgery? Radiation to the pelvic area? An injury involving your spine or your anus?

Be frank about your concerns. Although fecal incontinence is rarely the first sign of rectal cancer or another serious medical condition, let your doctor know about your fears. And make sure the doctor knows exactly how the incontinence is affecting your life and how you are attempting to manage it. During your evaluation, your physician—or a nurse who specializes in incontinence—may be able to suggest more effective ways to manage the problem.

Physical exam

A physical examination is an important part of the diagnostic process but does not provide a definite answer in about one-third of patients. Often, further tests are necessary (see "Testing," at right).

During the physical examination, your clinician will check your reflexes, walking gait, and senses for signs of general neurological disease or damage. He or she will also examine your abdomen for signs of bowel problems. The main difference in an evaluation for fecal incontinence is that the rectal exam is more thorough than usual.

First, the clinician looks at and inside the anus for any skin damage or scarring from previous injuries or medical procedures. The shape of your anus—whether open or closed, perfectly round or asymmetrical, intact or cracked—is noted. Using a Q-tip or pinprick, the doctor touches various points around your anus to see if it puckers up—a normal "winking" reflex.

Next, the doctor inserts a gloved finger into your rectum for the digital rectal exam (DRE) to feel for the presence of hemorrhoids, growths, tears, protrusions, or scars. You may be asked to squeeze your muscles around the doctor's finger or to bear down as if you were straining to have a bowel movement. The doctor may be able to feel whether the puborectalis muscle in your pelvic floor is working to keep the colon and rectum at the proper angle. If you feel any pain during the exam, tell the physician.

Testing

After your physical, you may be scheduled for additional tests.

Laboratory tests

If the doctor suspects an infection is causing diarrhea, he or she may take a stool sample and have it cultured in the laboratory so it can be examined for bacteria or other microbes. Other laboratory tests may be used to rule out various conditions that can have fecal incontinence as a symptom.

Exams using scopes

The doctor may want to use a scope to take a closer look at the area suspected of causing the problem. Using a viewing device, your physician can check for tumors, inflammation, prolapse, or other changes in the lining of your lower colon or rectum that might indicate damage to underlying nerves and muscles.

■ **Flexible sigmoidoscopy.** This test can be performed in your physician's office or in the hospital. You'll receive instructions in advance on how to clean out your bowels—usually by fasting and taking a laxative the night before the test and using an enema an hour or two before your appointment. While you lie on your side, the doctor inserts a lubricated sigmoidoscope (a flexible scope about half an inch wide and two feet long) through your rectum into your colon. The scope has a light and video camera, along with mechanisms for adding air or washing the area to get a better view. The exam takes about 20 minutes.

Colonoscopy. Using this method, the doctor examines the full length of the colon. This method is often used to screen for colon polyps and other signs of colon cancer. The test requires sedation. It is usually not necessary to evaluate fecal incontinence, but it may be suggested if colorectal cancer is suspected or if screening might be advisable for other reasons.

Other scope exams. For an examination that does not include the colon, your physician may use a proctoscope to examine the rectum or an anoscope to view the anal canal only.

Other tests

Even if nothing is apparent on the clinical exam and you don't recall a difficult childbirth or other trauma, your doctor may still suspect that your anal sphincters are damaged. The following tests can help determine whether that is the case.

Anorectal manometry. A doctor may use this test to measure the pressure inside your rectum and anal sphincters. After you have an enema, the clinician inserts into your rectum a small flexible tube (about the width of a rectal thermometer). The tube has a deflated balloon at the end. As you rest, squeeze, and bear down, the pressure inside your rectum and inside each sphincter is recorded on a polygraph-like display. This testing helps the clinician assess the strength of your sphincters and determine whether they are relaxing and constricting at the proper times. The test is a little bit like urodynamic testing (see page 10) for urinary incontinence.

Endoanal ultrasound. This technique, also known as endoanal sonography, uses sound waves, rather than x-rays, to create images of the internal and external anal sphincters. Inserting a slim ultrasound probe into the anus, the physician should be able to see how your sphincter muscles move and determine whether any portions of the muscles are missing or have become too thin. It is important to distinguish incontinence caused by sphincter damage—which may be surgically repairable—from that caused by other muscle or nerve damage. Endoanal sonography can help distinguish who will benefit from surgery and who will best respond to nonsurgical approaches.

Anorectal electromyography (EMG). This test helps assess whether your muscles are contracting and relaxing appropriately. For an anal sphincter EMG, the doctor inserts a small electrode-containing sponge into your anal canal. The sponge records electrical signals from the sphincter muscles as you squeeze and relax.

Pudendal nerve terminal motor latency. This technique helps assess whether your nerves are properly able to control the action of your anal sphincters. For a pudendal nerve study, the clinician does a digital rectal exam with a small electrode attached. The doctor delivers a mild electrical current to the pudendal nerve and measures the amount of time it takes for the sphincter to contract in response to the current.

Magnetic resonance imaging (MRI). Rarely, as an alternative to ultrasound, some physicians use MRI to examine their patients' sphincters. However, the images produced by MRI are not nearly as revealing as ultrasound images. MRI uses magnetic fields and radio waves to create cross-sectional images.

X-rays. Rarely, special x-rays may be taken to help evaluate the anatomy and functioning of your pelvic floor muscles and rectum, or to locate any obstruction in the colon. These exams go by different names: defecography, dynamic defecography, or evacuation proctography. Before your appointment, you clean out your colon as you would for flexible sigmoidoscopy (see page 36). One hour before the exam, you may be asked to drink some barium solution.

Just before the exam, a technician will insert a substance with the consistency of stool that is visible on x-ray into your rectum. Then the technician takes x-ray video images as you cough, squeeze your buttocks, strain, and defecate on a special commode. This test may reveal abnormal positioning of the rectum or relaxation of sphincter muscles. The exam is not painful, but you may have an uncomfortable feeling of needing to have a bowel movement.

Treating fecal incontinence

Fecal incontinence can be treated. It is up to you and your doctor to decide which treatment is best for you. Choices range from dietary changes and bowel training regimens to surgery. The approach you select will depend on the cause and severity of the condition. To help you gain the best possible control, physicians often recommend a combination of approaches. In most cases, treatment begins with nonsurgical options.

Diet and medication

The good news is that your diet can have a major impact on your bowel function by changing the consistency of the stool and the predictability of your bowel movements. That means there are potentially beneficial changes that you can make, such as eating more fiber or eliminating foods that irritate your system. Depending on your symptoms, your doctor may suggest diet changes to improve bowel control or make your condition easier to manage.

Virtually everyone can derive some benefit from dietary changes. For example, people with sphincter problems can gain better control by taking steps to eliminate diarrhea. Symptoms of irritable bowel syndrome can be helped by identifying and eliminating specific irritating foods.

Quick tip

One of the easiest and most effective ways to reduce fecal leakage is to take a fiber supplement, such as Metamucil, Konsyl, or Citrucel, daily. These products, found in any drugstore, work to control both constipation and diarrhea by absorbing water into the stool and creating large, soft, easy-to-pass stool. Make sure to drink plenty of liquid with the fiber supplement so as to avoid constipation. It may seem counterintuitive, but drinking plenty of water with the fiber supplement also helps control diarrhea because the fiber absorbs the water and prevents leakage of watery stool.

Controlling diarrhea

Diarrhea is a very common aggravating factor in fecal incontinence. If you tend to have loose stools, you may be able to make them firmer and easier to control by adding fiber to your diet or by taking a bulking agent or fiber supplement (see "Quick tip," at left). High-fiber diets can be helpful for both constipation and diarrhea. Dietary fiber can absorb up to 30 times its weight in water. It produces formed but soft stools, and may "normalize" your bowels. Good sources of dietary fiber are bran cereals, uncooked fruits and vegetables, whole-grain breads and pasta, and brown rice.

Specific foods may trigger diarrhea in some people. The National Institute of Diabetes and Digestive and Kidney Diseases (NIDDK) has identified a number of foods you might try eliminating from your diet to see if your symptoms improve (see "Foods that may cause diarrhea," page 39). According to the NIDDK, potential sources of trouble include caffeine, cured or smoked meats, spicy foods, alcohol, dairy products, fruits, fatty and greasy foods, and some sweeteners (such as sorbitol, xylitol, mannitol, and fructose) that are found in many diet drinks, fruit drinks, sugarless gum, and candies.

Your physician may advise a change in the medications you take for other conditions, in case they are contributing to diarrhea and incontinence problems. As an example, the antidiabetic drug metformin (Glucophage) sometimes causes chronic diarrhea, long after you start taking the drug. Orlistat (Xenical), a medication used to treat obesity, decreases the absorption of fat from the digestive tract. Side effects may include several distressing bowel symptoms, including oily seepage from the rectum, fecal urgency, and, for a few people, fecal incontinence.

If food seems to move through your digestive system rapidly, your doctor may suggest an antidiarrheal medicine such as loperamide (Imodium) or diphenoxylate and atropine (Lomotil). This can solid-

> **Foods that may cause diarrhea**
>
> Try eliminating or reducing the foods listed below, doing so one at a time for several days each, to determine whether one of them might be causing diarrhea.
>
> - cured or smoked meats
> - spicy foods
> - fatty and greasy foods
> - fruits
> - dairy products
> - alcohol
> - caffeine
> - sweeteners (sorbitol, xylitol, mannitol, fructose)

ify your stools and make them less frequent. Loperamide has the side benefit of increasing muscle tone in the internal anal sphincter, which can also help with incontinence. Another medication, the tricyclic antidepressant amitriptyline, also reduces the number of bowel movements. Some doctors have used it successfully to improve fecal incontinence, although the effectiveness of this treatment has not yet been confirmed in a controlled study.

Managing constipation

If your fecal incontinence is related to constipation, your health professional may suggest ways to train yourself to have regularly timed bowel movements. These may include increasing your fiber and fluid intake and using various stimuli (from a warm drink to an enema) to encourage a bowel movement at set times.

Pelvic muscle exercises and biofeedback

Using exercise to strengthen the muscles of the pelvic floor, including the anal sphincters, is a commonly recommended treatment for people with fecal incontinence. The studies evaluating the effectiveness of pelvic muscle training in treating fecal incontinence have shown inconsistent results. However, for people whose incontinence is less than severe and who prefer a self-help method to surgery, pelvic floor strengthening is worth trying. Combining this technique with dietary changes (increased fiber) and adjustment in medications as needed may improve the likelihood of success. As with any muscle-strengthening program, pelvic muscle strength begins to diminish as soon as the exercises are discontinued.

These exercises require some training, and biofeedback is an effective way to help identify the correct muscles and learn how to do the exercises correctly. Biofeedback training can help fecal incontinence in two ways. First, it helps you strengthen and coordinate the action of your sphincter muscles. Second, it can improve your ability to sense the presence of stool in the rectum.

If the biofeedback session is aimed at strengthening your pelvic muscles, the practitioner will insert a slim sensor into your rectum. (In women, it is sometimes placed in the vagina, or an additional sensor may be used there.) Other electrodes will be placed on your abdomen to help record muscle contractions there. A computer screen provides feedback about the strength of your contractions and about whether you are using the correct muscles.

If the biofeedback training is aimed at improving your ability to sense stool in the rectum, the practitioner will use anorectal manometry equipment to vary the pressure in your rectum. This is intended to increase the sensitivity of the rectum, which, in turn, helps some patients to recognize the presence of stool before the situation becomes desperate.

Whether biofeedback will help depends on the cause and severity of your incontinence and your ability to learn and practice the exercises. The improvements may only be modest. But biofeedback and exercise are so safe they are almost always recommended before more invasive treatments.

■ **Pelvic muscle conditioning without exercise.** Another form of biofeedback training uses electrical stimulation (see page 19). As a part of this treatment, a small electrical shock is delivered to the anal sphincter, in hopes of bulking up the muscles. Unlike other biofeedback methods, electrical stimulation does the work for you. The concept is that the electrical stimulation produces much more muscle activity than patients can accomplish themselves, even with standard biofeedback. There are several reports that suggest this may be of value. But, so far, there have been no controlled studies that have described its effectiveness in comparison with biofeedback or no treatment.

Surgical treatments

If you do require surgery, the exact approach will depend on the cause of your symptoms and your response to previous treatments. Some of these approaches have been around for years—although the techniques are always being modified and updated to improve results. Other approaches are more recent developments.

Sacral nerve stimulation (SNS)

Sacral nerve stimulation is a minimally invasive approach with a low rate of medical complications. For this procedure, the surgeon inserts a kind of pacemaker to provide continuous electric stimulation to the anal sphincter to keep it closed. Also called sacral neuromodulation, this technique has long been used for urinary incontinence (see "Sacral neuromodulation," page 23) and has only more recently been adapted for fecal incontinence as well.

In 2011, the FDA approved the use of this procedure for fecal incontinence based on encouraging results from medical studies, including a 2010 study of 133 patients published in *Annals of Surgery*. Among the patients in this study, episodes of fecal incontinence decreased from about nine per week before surgery to about two per week a full year after surgery, and three per week two years after surgery.

Overlapping sphincteroplasty

If your anal sphincter was damaged during childbirth, anal surgery, or other trauma, your physician may suggest a sphincteroplasty to repair it. The external anal sphincter forms a ring around the anus. If there is a breach or interruption in the ring of muscle, you may not be able to close it tightly enough to keep stool in. During a sphincteroplasty, the surgeon will reattach the damaged ends and stitch them together to create a complete ring of muscle. This restores the anus to its proper shape. Sphincteroplasty has been used for decades and is the most common surgery used to treat fecal incontinence. It is very safe. However, the effectiveness of sphincteroplasty may vary for different kinds of patients. Therefore, careful evaluation before surgery is important.

While you are healing from sphincteroplasty, you may have discomfort, bruising, and swelling in the wound area. Wound infections sometimes happen after sphincteroplasty—as they do after all surgeries in the anorectal area. As with any surgery, you should be scrupulous in following your doctor's instructions on cleaning and caring for the wound.

Sphincteroplasty has been shown to be successful—at least initially—in up to 75% of patients with severe fecal incontinence. However, there have also been discouraging reports about deterioration in function over time. In two studies, about half of the patients who underwent this treatment said they were experiencing some urinary or fecal incontinence, had required further surgery, or had developed other bowel problems, when contacted four to 12 years later.

If incontinence is still a problem after the surgery, your surgeon may recommend additional biofeedback. In fact, some surgeons suggest it for all patients as soon as the wound is healed, in order to maximize the chance of a good outcome.

Rectal prolapse repair

One common cause of fecal incontinence is rectal prolapse—the dropping of the rectum because of muscle weakness. If it is not treated, this condition can cause permanent damage to the sphincter. If it is surgically repaired, however, fecal incontinence may become much less severe, and, in many cases, it will be entirely cured. This surgery is most successful if done early, so don't put off reporting your symptoms to your doctor.

There are a variety of surgical options for treating rectal prolapse. The particular option that you are offered will be based on—among other things—your health. In general, younger, healthier patients will be offered an operation that involves an abdominal incision and removal of part of the bowel. This surgery can be done either through a traditional open incision or by using laparoscopy (a camera-aided surgery that leaves a very small scar). In general, older patients will be offered a simpler surgery, through the anus. In this case, the protruding rectal tissue will simply be cut off, so it does not stretch the anal sphincter. Both surgeries work well in the short term. However, an abdominal approach is generally preferable, if possible, because it lasts longer.

Artificial sphincter

An artificial bowel sphincter is the only surgical option available in the United States for patients whose severe sphincter injury is beyond repair or does not respond to other surgery. This procedure was approved by the FDA in 2001. It is best performed in younger, healthier patients.

The doctor inserts an artificial device that circles the anal sphincter. It keeps the anus closed until the patient squeezes a control pump to open it. The opening, in turn, allows a bowel movement to pass. Afterward, the cuff gradually closes. For a male patient, the control pump is implanted in the scrotum. For a female patient, it is inserted in the labium.

In follow-up studies, the implantation of an artificial sphincter cured fecal incontinence, and significantly improved quality of life, in most patients. But some patients required repeat surgery or had complications, such as infection; these patients had to have the device removed.

The surgery is not recommended unless you have the manual dexterity to work the pump. Also, once the device is implanted, you will not be able to deliver a baby vaginally or engage in anal intercourse, either of which could damage the cuff.

Dynamic graciloplasty

Dynamic graciloplasty is a rarely used technique that has not yet been approved by the FDA, although it is more often performed in Europe. It may be effective if a patient's sphincter is damaged and if there is also nerve damage to the anus. In this case, the surgeon wraps a piece of the gracilis muscle (from the inner thigh) around the anus to substitute for the damaged sphincter. The surgeon then implants a kind of pacemaker, similar to a sacral nerve stimulator (see page 40). This keeps the newly created muscle closed and prevents stool from leaking out.

This technique has some reported complications, including constipation as well as pain and swelling in the thigh from which the muscle is obtained. However, in one U.S. report, researchers found that patients showed a significant improvement in the extent of incontinence and in their quality of life although incontinence was not completely cured. Two years after this surgery, patients needed half as many pads to control their incontinence. The number of incontinent episodes involving solid stool dropped from 9.3 to 1.3 per week. And those involving liquid were reduced from 9.1 to 3.5.

Colostomy

A final surgical technique—usually done as a last resort—is colostomy. This means that feces are entirely diverted from the rectum and anal canal and instead leave the body through a surgically created opening. In a colostomy, the surgeon attaches the end of the bowel to an opening made in the patient's abdomen. The surgery is performed under general anesthesia and requires several days of hospitalization.

After a colostomy, you will need to care for the opening on the skin (called the ostomy), and you will need to wear a small pouch outside your body to collect waste material. Modern ostomy bags are not visible when you are dressed, and they control odor very effectively. Most of the time, no one is even aware that you have had the surgery.

Injection of bulking agents

Thus far, the injection of bulking agents to tighten the sphincter has not seen the success that had been hoped for. In situations of minor incontinence, small beads of carbon or silicon can be placed between the internal and external sphincters. The beads thicken the overall sphincter complex with the goal of keeping it closed. The surgery is simple and is usually done in an office setting. But its effectiveness, particularly over the long term, has not met expectations.

Managing fecal incontinence

Even if medical treatment doesn't fully alleviate your symptoms, it is likely to diminish them and make your condition more manageable. You can reclaim a sense of control by learning some management techniques and being prepared in advance should an accident occur. Seek help from health professionals, such as continence nurses, and support organizations, such as the International Foundation for Functional Gastrointestinal Disorders (www.iffgd.org).

Skin care

When the skin comes in contact with fecal material for a length of time, it can become irritated and inflamed. As a result, proper care of the skin in the anal area is essential to maintaining comfort and preventing skin deterioration. Skin irritation is more than a misery. It can invite infection and even compromise your treatment if the skin becomes too sore for your muscles to work well. If you have both urinary and fecal incontinence, bacteria in the feces can react with urine to produce ammonia, which lowers the skin pH and leaves it more vulnerable to infection. Yeast infections can also develop, when yeast in the feces is nurtured by contact with urine.

Skin should be cleansed after each episode of incontinence. Choose an extremely mild, nonalkaline soap—such as Dove or Basis—or buy one of the special cleansers designed to gently dissolve and remove stool and urine. These are nonirritating, soap-free cleansing lotions; some are available in portable disposable wipes. They eliminate the need to scrub areas of tender skin, and some do not require that you rinse the skin after use. In studies conducted in nursing homes, the cleansers worked better than soap to prevent breakdown of sensitive perineal skin in patients with incontinence. After cleansing, allow the area to air-dry if possible, or blow dry with a hair dryer set on cool, or pat it dry (don't rub). Afterward, apply a protective moisturizer or moisture barrier to protect the skin from damage by urine or stool contact. Barrier products such as petroleum jelly, Aquaphor, or Desitin are readily available and inexpensive.

Film-forming skin protectants—applied by spray, applicator, or individual wipe—go on as a liquid but rapidly evaporate. They leave behind a film of clear acrylate. This barrier allows airflow, but protects the skin from moisture. Film-forming skin protectants may help reduce the rubbing of pads or absorbent products or make it less irritating to use products applied with adhesive. Some films last as long as three days before reapplication is needed.

To treat or protect against fungal infection, you may be instructed to use an ointment or cream containing an antifungal agent, such as clotrimazole or miconazole. Ask whether you should apply another barrier product while using the antifungal.

A nurse who deals with incontinence or stoma care can offer advice on skin care issues. For more

Figure 9 Prevalence of fecal incontinence according to age and sex

This chart compares fecal incontinence in men and women in each age group in Australia in 2002. Some newer 2008 statistics are available for women in the United States (see page 33), but not for men.
Reprinted with permission from Medical Journal of Australia, *Jan. 21, 2002, pp. 54–57.*

information, go to the Web site of the National Association for Continence at www.nafc.org.

Reducing odor

Minimizing the odor of stool can make leakage less noticeable to yourself and others. Dietary changes can help by eliminating foods that commonly increase stool odor. Such foods include fish, eggs, asparagus, garlic, cruciferous vegetables (such as cabbage, broccoli, and cauliflower), onions, beans, and turnips.

Odor can also be reduced by taking an internal deodorant containing chlorophyllin copper (such as Nullo) or bismuth subgallate (such as Devrom). Both are available without prescription. However, chlorophyllin may color your urine and stool green. This creates the possibility of "grass-stained" clothing if an accident occurs. If cramping or diarrhea occurs when taking chlorophyllin, reduce the dose. If symptoms continue, stop taking it.

Containment and collection options

Absorbent products, such as pads and disposable undergarments, are designed primarily for urinary incontinence, and people with fecal incontinence often find them unsatisfactory. Of the range of choices available (see "Managing urinary incontinence," page 29), those that provide "heavy" protection are most likely to be helpful for fecal incontinence. According to the limited studies available, disposable products with super-absorbent materials may provide the best protection and be easiest on your skin.

There are also fecal collection devices (such as Bard FCD and Hollister), which are pouches that adhere to the skin around the anus to collect uncontrolled stool leakage. These devices control stool odor and can drain off liquid into a separate bag. You can order such products through a medical supply house or catalog.

Anal plugs contain fecal incontinence by blocking the passage of stool. Limited research on these devices suggests that they are not always easy to live with. However, they can be an effective primary or occasional management technique for some people. Devices made of polyurethane (such as Peristeen) seem to perform better than those made of polyvinyl alcohol. Anal plugs are primarily used by people with diminished anal sensation and those with significant neurological impairment from injury or illness.

Enemas and suppositories

Some people with fecal incontinence are able to eliminate or minimize incontinence or soiling by using enemas or suppositories each morning to cleanse feces from their rectum and lower colon. You should seek medical advice about your choice of enema or suppository, and about the advisability of using this approach.

Emotional concerns

Gaining control over fecal incontinence is a psychological as well as physical challenge. The emotional repercussions can be very difficult to handle. You may find it helpful to remind yourself that this is a very common medical condition. Many other people, like you, are coping with the same condition, as the result of surgery, childbirth, or medical illness.

If you have lived with the problem for a long time before seeking help, it may take time and professional support for you to address your painful feelings and regain confidence in your ability to fully participate in normal activities and relationships.

Help is available from health professionals, therapists, and support groups. You can benefit greatly from the advice and experiences of others with the same problem, whether through informal contact or a support group. Most importantly, remember that yours is a medical condition, not a personal weakness.

Resources

Organizations

American Physical Therapy Association
1111 N. Fairfax St.
Alexandria, VA 22314
800-999-2782 (toll-free)
www.apta.org

This organization can recommend physical therapists trained in pelvic floor exercise and therapy.

American Society of Colon and Rectal Surgeons
85 W. Algonquin Road, Suite 550
Arlington Heights, IL 60005
847-290-9184
www.fascrs.org

This professional society offers educational materials on fecal incontinence and many bowel-related tests and procedures. The Web site includes a locator for certified colorectal surgeons.

American Urogynecologic Society
2025 M St. NW, Suite 800
Washington, DC 20036
202-367-1167
www.mypelvichealth.org

This professional society offers educational materials on incontinence and advice on locating a urogynecologist. The Web site includes a locator for member urogynecologists, nurse practitioners, and physical therapists.

American Urological Association
1000 Corporate Blvd.
Linthicum, MD 21090
866-746-4282 (toll-free)
www.urologyhealth.org

This professional society provides patient information on urologic disease and a doctor-locator function on its Web site.

Biofeedback Certification International Alliance
10200 W. 44th Ave., Suite 310
Wheat Ridge, CO 80033
866-908-8713 (toll-free)
www.bcia.org

The Web site for this organization can help you identify certified biofeedback practitioners in your area, including those certified to treat elimination disorders and pelvic pain.

National Association for Continence
P.O. Box 1019
Charleston, SC 29402
800-252-3337 (toll-free)
www.nafc.org

The largest consumer advocacy and educational organization dealing with incontinence, NAFC provides a wide range of pamphlets and other materials, including a detailed brand-name resource guide to products, devices, and medications used to maintain an active life while coping with incontinence.

Wound, Ostomy, and Continence Nurses Society
15000 Commerce Parkway, Suite C
Mt. Laurel, NJ 08054
888-224-9626 (toll-free)
www.wocn.org

Many members of this professional society specialize in the management and treatment of urinary and fecal incontinence and related conditions.

Books

Managing and Treating Urinary Incontinence
Diane K. Newman, R.N.C.
(Health Professions Press, 2008)

Although written for health professionals, this book is readable and contains practical advice on managing urinary incontinence.

Regaining Bladder Control: What Every Woman Needs to Know
Rebecca G. Rogers, M.D., Janet Yagoda Shagam, Ph.D., and Shelley Kleinschmidt
(Prometheus Books, 2006)

This book provides supportive and practical information about getting help for urinary incontinence. Written by a urogynecologist in collaboration with medical writers, it includes several worksheets, questions to ask, and clear illustrations and photographs. There are chapters on fecal incontinence and prolapse.

Women's Waterworks: Curing Incontinence
Dr. Pauline Chiarelli
(Chiarelli Healthcare, 2007)

A short, practical, easy-to-read book of advice and information with illustrations.

Special Health Reports from Harvard Medical School

Women's Health: Fifty and Forward
Celeste Robb-Nicholson, M.D., and Beverly Merz
(Harvard Health Publications, 2010)

An overview of health issues that become more common as women pass age 50. The report covers both physical health and emotional health, and includes a special section on 10 steps to a longer, healthier life.

Living Longer, Living Better
Anne Fabiny, M.D., and Francesca Coltrera

This Special Health Report, for men and women, discusses diet, exercise, health screening, and other topics that can influence your overall health and longevity. The report includes a special section entitled "Can we extend healthy human life?"